LEAN IN 15

THE SHAPE PLAN

JOE WICKS

The Body Coach

First published 2016 by Bluebird
an imprint of Pan Macmillan
20 New Wharf Road, London N1 9RR
Associated companies throughout the world
www.panmacmillan.com

ISBN 978-1-5098-0069-8
Copyright © Joe Wicks 2016

Food photography © Maja Smend
Fitness photography in Chapter 6 and images on pages 4, 8–9, 22–3, 28–9, 72,
96–7, 147, 176–7, 194–5, 221, 222–33, 237 © Glen Burrows

The right of Joe Wicks to be identified as the author of this work has been asserted
by him in accordance with the Copyright, Designs and Patents Act 1988.

Grateful acknowledgement is made to 'My Lean Winners' and the 'Lean in 15 Heroes'
for permission to include the images on pages 225–33 and 238–9.

Credits
Publisher: Carole Tonkinson
Assistant Editor: Olivia Morris
Design: Ami Smithson
Desk Editor: Claire Gatzen
Food Photography: Maja Smend
Fitness Photography: Glen Burrows
Food Styling: Bianca Nice
Prop Styling: Lydia Brun

Pan Macmillan does not have any control over, or any responsibility for, any author
or third-party websites referred to in or on this book.

9 8 7 6 5 4 3

A CIP catalogue record for this book is available from the British Library.

Printed in Italy

Designed and Typeset by www.cabinlondon.co.uk

Visit www.panmacmillan.com to read more about all our books and to buy them.
You will also find features, author interviews and news of any author events, and you
can sign up for e-newsletters so that you're always first to hear about our new releases.

Bluebird publish inspirational lifestyle books, bringing you the
very latest in diet, self-help and popular psychology, as well as
parenting, career and business, and memoir.

We make books for life in every sense: life-enhancing but also
lasting; the ones you will turn to again and again for inspiration.

**For 10 extra Lean in 15 recipes and to hear more about
Bluebird visit** www.TheBodyCoachBooks.com

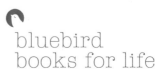

bluebird
books for life

CONTENTS

///////////////////////////////////////

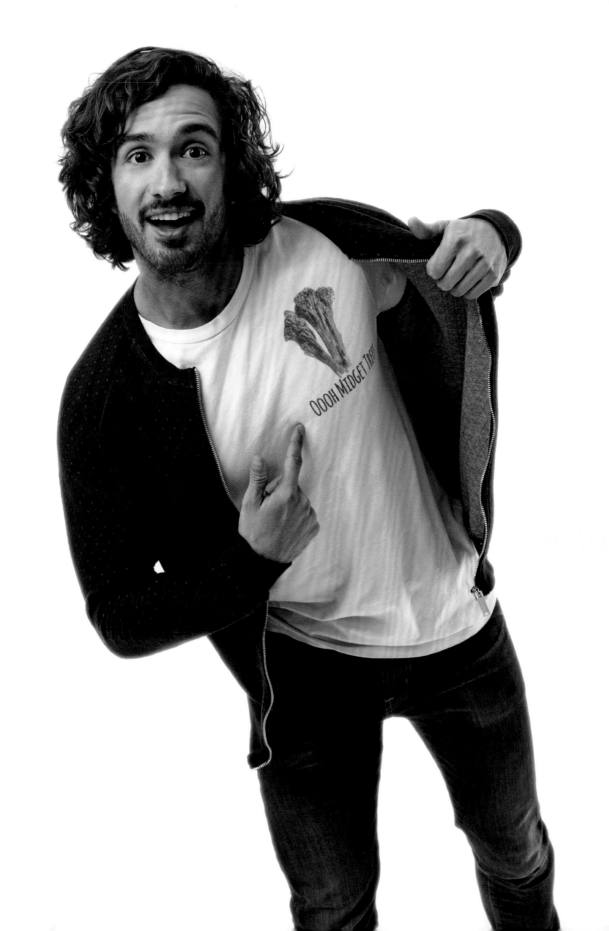

INTRODUCTION

//

Hello, you little winner, it's me again, Joe Wicks, The Body Coach. I'm back with another instalment of *Lean in 15* and this time it's *The Shape Plan*.

For those who haven't heard of Lean in 15, here's a quick recap. I used to be a personal trainer and boot camp owner in Surrey, UK. Then one day in January 2014, from my little flat in Surbiton, I had an idea.

I started to post 15-second videos on Instagram (@thebodycoach) showing people how to cook a lean and healthy meal in under 15 minutes. The #Leanin15 hashtag was born and my little idea has gone on to inspire and help hundreds of thousands of people all over the world to cook, exercise and get lean.

I've used the power of social media and my love of exercise and nutrition to share my message with the world, and now my mission continues with this second book in the Lean in 15 series.

My aim is always to keep things quick and simple because I know that life gets busy and we don't have time to spend hours in the kitchen every day. With Lean in 15 I'm going to show you that you can have a busy job and family life and still find the time to stay lean.

Book 1, *The Shift Plan*, was all about shifting unwanted body fat with my post-workout carbohydrate-refuel method and high intensity cardio sessions. This phase – the Shape Plan – is all about shaping the body by building lean muscle with resistance training.

> ❜ You can have a busy job and family life and still find the time to stay lean ❜

The four workouts are detailed with images and instructions in Chapter 6. These sessions will be challenging, as we combine weight training with HIIT cardio, but trust me, the results will be worth it. This tried and tested training system is currently transforming men and women all over the world. And don't worry, you don't need to start with Book 1. You can start to live the Lean in 15 lifestyle with this book.

The main focus in this book is on building strong, lean muscle while reducing body fat. By increasing your lean muscle mass, you will increase your metabolic rate. This means you can eat more of the food you love, burn more body fat and stay lean all year round.

Don't be put off by the thought of lifting weights. It's not going to make you look 'bulky' like some 1980s German body builder. No, no, no – that just doesn't happen in the real world. This plan is, however, going to teach you how to fuel your body and make you stronger, more defined and leaner than ever.

The great thing about the Shape Plan is that you really don't need an expensive gym membership or lots of costly equipment to complete the workouts. You can, of course, train at the gym but if you decide to train from home all you will need to invest in is a workout bench and a good set of dumbbells. And that's it! You can get to work on building the body you've always wanted.

As the training intensity builds, so too do the energy demands placed on your body, and this means that instead of having just one carbohydrate meal (as I recommend people do in *The Shift Plan*), you now get to smash three carb meals on a training day. Wooo wooo! Hello carbs. Get in my belly.

With Lean in 15 the days of going hungry and calorie counting are over. The days of standing on the sad step (the scales) and measuring your success by a number are gone. I'm here to show you that there is another way. The low-calorie diet industry has got it all wrong. The science is old. The fat-loss 'diet' products being constantly marketed to you are the reason people are struggling to lose body fat. Sorry for the little rant but it really does upset me! I literally scream at the TV when I see adverts for new diet pills, dust diets or one of those drinks that they claim expand in the stomach to make you feel fuller. How can they even get away with that on TV?

The simple truth is this – nutrition doesn't need to be complicated. You don't need to starve yourself to get lean. You don't need to deprive yourself of lovely tasty foods and eat like a rabbit to burn fat. And you really don't need to spend your life feeling helpless and unconfident in your body because you've tried and failed on every diet.

Lean in 15 is different because it's not a diet. It's a flexible approach that will fit into your life and become a lifestyle. Diets have an end date but this does not, which is why it works for so many people. This book will provide a mini-education in nutrition, where you will learn the basics and follow a simple plan to take control and build a strong, healthy body.

Is it going to be easy? No, of course it's not. Not at first, at least. Changing habits is really challenging. If it was easy everybody would be walking around looking super-lean all year. It's going to take a lot of meal prep and effort in the kitchen. It's going to take real dedication and consistency with your training, but when you see the results and grow in confidence and fitness every week it will be worth every single bit of grub, sweat and skipped beer. The hardest part is actually starting, but once you do you'll love it and momentum will carry you all the way to lean land.

The principles of the Shape Plan are taken from my 90 Day Shift, Shape and Sustain programme which has changed the lives of hundreds of thousands of people all over the world. I've included a few transformations and testimonials in this book but if you want to see more and get inspired please visit thebodycoach.co.uk.

So here's to the new school. To a new challenge and a new way of doing things. Take this book and run with it. Commit to making a few small lifestyle changes and it will transform your body and the way you eat forever.

I'd like to say a big thank you for picking up and investing in this book. I really hope you find the information useful and enjoy the recipes I've worked hard to create. You are in control of the way you look and feel, so go and make yourself a lean winner.

Keep it Lean.

Joe Wicks

> **' NUTRITION DOESN'T NEED TO BE COMPLICATED. YOU DON'T NEED TO STARVE YOURSELF TO GET LEAN '**

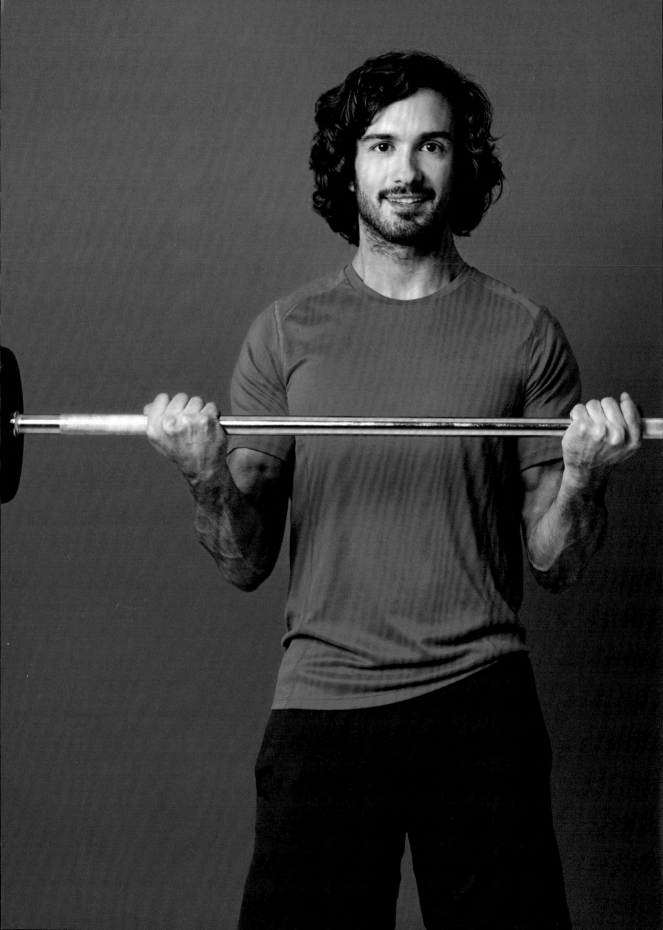

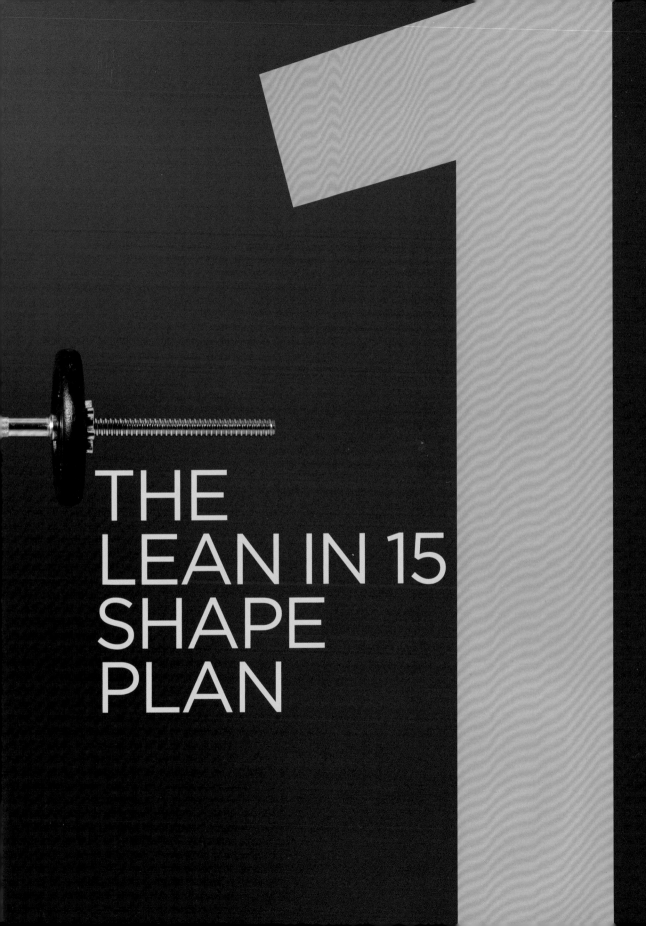

THE
LEAN IN 15
SHAPE
PLAN

WHAT MAKES LEAN IN 15 DIFFERENT?

//

Before we get started I think it's really important to remind ourselves exactly why low-calorie diets don't work in the long term. Let's just think about how many diets have been and gone in the past years. I'm sure you can reel off a few from the top of your head and may have even tried some of them yourself. Was it fun? Probably not. Could you imagine spending your whole life on it? Errrm, no way! And that's the problem. You should never start something that you know you won't enjoy or be able to stick with.

Low-calorie diets have one thing in common – they are unsustainable. This is because they rely on deprivation and they are both mentally and physically draining. People can't live their lives on a diet that makes them feel hungry, unhappy, low on energy and obsessed by the numbers on a set of scales.

Many diets also fail to educate people on nutrition and instead focus on creating a huge calorie deficit. This is an outdated approach and doesn't focus on health at all. For example, some diets ban all foods high in fat. So eating an avocado, which is full of heart-healthy monounsaturated fats, is suddenly a sin and banned! This doesn't make sense as we know that not all

'Low-calorie diets have one thing in common – they are unsustainable'

fats are the same, and some fats such as omega-3s are actually essential to the body. What's even more frustrating is seeing those same diet companies promote and sell highly processed low-fat junk foods with zero nutritional value to the body.

This is why things need to change. Education is key to long-term health. A calorie is not just a calorie. Your body absorbs and processes fat from an avocado very differently to hydrogenated fat from a doughnut or microwaveable ready meal. Lean in 15 is all about eating for energy and health, which is why I want to educate you on macronutrients (more on that in a bit!) so that you learn to eat for now and for the future, and you and your whole family stay lean.

Yes, those crash diets may seem appealing a month before your holiday because they will make you burn fat at the beginning, but let's think about the body as an engine and your food as the fuel. If you drop your calories really low, really fast – for example, to 1,000 calories per day, as some diets suggest – then, yes, your engine will turn to stored fat for fuel. But the body is very smart and adapts quickly to conserve energy. If your body thinks you're not going to fuel it for a long time, then anything you do feed it is going to be stored and the body will start to down-regulate (slow down) any non-essential processes (such as burning fat and building new muscle). This results in a loss of lean muscle tissue, which decreases your metabolism – which is the last thing you want happening.

A low-calorie life is an unhappy life

When your body stops burning fat on 1,000 kcal a day, where can you go from there? Do you drop to 900, 800, 700 per day? Before you know it you're in a position where your body cannot burn fat and has no chance whatsoever of building lean muscle tissue. You'll have no energy, you'll be miserable, your immune system will be weakened and your hair, skin and nails will suffer. Prolonged low-calorie dieting can also affect your thyroid gland and the hormones in your body, which makes fat loss even harder.

I want you to throw all those diet books away. You don't need to struggle any more and obsess over counting calories. Your body is an engine and your aim should always be to get it burning fat while fuelling it with as much food as possible. This way, your life

> ❛ LEAN IN 15 IS ALL ABOUT EATING FOR ENERGY AND HEALTH ❜

can be happy and full of energy, and if you do hit a fat-loss plateau you can make small adjustments to reignite your fat-burning.

Understanding your body a bit more

I really want you to understand from the start that your body is unique. So many diets out there have a 'one size fits all' approach to fat loss and just assume that everyone is the same. For example, that all women need to eat 1,200 kcal a day to lose weight and all males 1,600 kcal. This couldn't be further from the truth as everyone has different energy demands and metabolic rates.

Individuals also respond differently to certain food groups and ways of eating, so it's really important that you listen to your body. There is no right or wrong when it comes to your nutrition and I want you to challenge yourself to try things out and establish how your body runs best and on what fuel.

This is the reason I create tailored online meal plans and put all of my clients through a 'bio feedback' process. It's a simple technique, unique to my plan, whereby in cycle one I put people on a reduced-carbohydrate diet for 4 weeks. During this time, they eat only one post-workout meal with carbs. Then in cycle two, the Shape Plan, I increase their carb intake to three carb meals on a training day and reduce their fat intake, which allows the client to get essential feedback on their body based on their nutrition (for example, their energy levels, sleep patterns, digestion, food sensitivities and emotional imbalances). Without this testing period some people may never find out just how to fuel their body optimally.

With the recipes and workouts in this book, you can begin to do the same thing at home today. Trust your instincts and take notes on your progress. If you're feeling sluggish on the days you eat three carb meals, you might want to go back to one carb meal a day (as recommended in *The Shift Plan*). If the recipes feel like too much food or not enough, listen to your body and adjust accordingly. You should eat to feel awesome all day, every day. If you are energized from the inside out, you will live a happier and more productive life and find staying lean and healthy much easier.

Why don't you list the calories on recipes?

I have chosen not to list the calorie or macro content of the meals in this book as I want you to get away from numbers-based

> ‘ Trust your instincts and take notes on your progress ,

thinking and start to gauge your own energy demands and portion sizes. I don't want you to think that the portions in my recipes are the Holy Grail for your fat loss. If you feel they are either too small or too big you can adjust them to ensure that your body is being fuelled properly on both a training day and a rest day. The key here is to listen to your body, don't go hungry, and make small adjustments when you need to.

Let's have a quick lesson on metabolism so that you understand a bit more about your body and how it works from an energy perspective.

Resting metabolic rate (RMR)

Resting metabolic rate is the energy required by your body to stay alive with no activity at complete rest. This literally means the energy (kcal) needed to breathe and function while lying down asleep. Consider this your base level or the minimum energy required by your body each day for breathing, blood circulation, controlling body temperature, cell growth, and brain and nerve function. Your resting metabolic rate accounts for around 70 per cent of your daily energy expenditure. This isn't taking into account any exercise and activity you do.

This number is different for everyone and is not static. Various factors such as age, sex, weight, height and fat-free body mass determine your RMR. Lean muscle tissue is more metabolically active than body fat, meaning it requires more energy. So, put simply, the leaner you are, the more food you can enjoy. This means your goal should always be to increase or maintain a good level of lean body mass. And that is what the Shape Plan is all about.

Crash dieting is something that has been shown to reduce RMR, which is why as soon as people come off a low-calorie diet and start eating more food, they often regain the weight very fast. Not only this but they then struggle even more to lose that body fat again.

Low-calorie dieting = bad
Building lean muscle = good!

Total daily energy expenditure

As well as your RMR, your body requires energy for physical activity. Total daily energy expenditure quantifies the total number

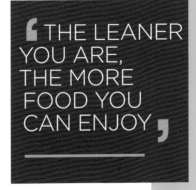

' THE LEANER YOU ARE, THE MORE FOOD YOU CAN ENJOY ,

of calories you burn in a day including your RMR and physical activity. This number will change daily depending on how active you are but accounts for all activity, such as getting out of bed, walking to work or doing a training session. But don't overthink this and start counting your steps and your calories in and out every day – that's not what you need to focus on. All you need to do is begin to be aware of your energy output and learn to eat in line with your energy demands. For example, if you are physically active in your job and train 5 days per week you will require more energy than someone who is sedentary in their job and exercises only twice a week. If you're super-active, you probably won't want to cut down the portions at all and may want to increase them.

Let's learn the basics of nutrition!

Hopefully that all made sense and you can now see just how important it is to fuel your body correctly, especially as you become more physically active. No more calorie counting for you! From this point on, you're going to respect your body with exercise, and you're going to love it with food.

Remember, a calorie is not just a calorie. That 'calories in vs calories out' rule does not focus on health. It's old science and old thinking. The simple fact is that the body digests and utilizes different foods in different ways, and I'll explain how.

We get our energy from three sources, called macronutrients. These are fats, proteins and carbohydrates. This is the fuel your body needs to survive, build, repair and grow. With the Shape Plan you will be eating all three of these macronutrients in the right ratios at the right time to ensure your body is burning fat and building lean muscle.

Just in case you haven't read my first book, I'll give you the quick lowdown on macronutrients and why they all have an important role to play.

Fats

Poor old fats seem to have a bad rep when it comes to fat loss. They often get thrown into one group and labelled as the bad guys. Hence my good mate the avocado being banned by some diets. But not all fats are the same. Some are good, some are

> **You're going to respect your body with exercise, and you're going to love it with food**

bad and some are absolutely essential to the body and must be obtained from the diet. Let's have a quick look at the different types of fat and their sources.

The three types of fat

There are three types of fat – saturated, monounsaturated and polyunsaturated. These are made up of chains of fatty acids which are different in structure.

It is important to note, though, that all fats contain a combination of different fatty acids. Therefore, no fat is pure saturated fat, or pure monounsaturated or polyunsaturated fat.

Saturated fat

Found in animal products such as eggs, butter, milk, cream, cheese and meat. This is the one we have been told is unhealthy by doctors for years due to its association with increased cholesterol and risk of coronary heart disease. This now very old, inaccurate research was based on studies using animals and not humans. It was also flawed because it focused only on total cholesterol which included both bad (LDL) and good (HDL) cholesterol. New research, however, has shown that saturated fat can actually increase the good cholesterol needed by the body, so it really isn't something you need to fear any more. Eat saturated fats in moderation, combine them with other types of fats and always try to get them from grass-fed animals.

Monounsaturated fat

Found in nuts, seeds, avocados and extra virgin olive oil. This type of fat is considered heart healthy because it increases the body's HDL cholesterol. This has been associated with a lower risk of heart disease and stroke, so aim to get this type of fat in your diet each day.

Polyunsaturated fat

Found in oily fish such as salmon and mackerel, and also flaxseeds and walnut oil. This fat can help lower your LDL cholesterol and is considered anti-inflammatory. It can also contain those all-important omega-3 fatty acids. Your body cannot produce polyunsaturated fats itself, so you must obtain them from your diet. My advice is to try to consume these at least three times per week.

So what's all this about inflammation then?

Inflammation is essential for our survival. It helps protect the body against infection and disease. Too much inflammation, however, is a bad thing and can lead to heart disease, diabetes, Alzheimer's and many types of cancer.

Omega-6s are considered pro-inflammatory while omega-3s are considered anti-inflammatory. A diet high in omega-6 but low in omega-3 increases inflammation, which is a bad thing. Therefore, it's essential that you get the right balance between omegas 3 and 6.

My top tips:

- Avoid cooking with sunflower oil, corn oil and vegetable oils, which are high in omega-6.
- Cook with coconut oil and butter from grass-fed animals instead.
- Cut down on processed foods, ready meals and fast food, which contain high amounts of omega-6.
- Aim to consume more wild-caught oily fish such as salmon.
- Try to eat grass-fed animals where possible.
- Get flaxseeds and chia seeds into your diet (add these to soups, smoothies, porridge and anything else you fancy).

Fats have various important roles:

1. Fat-soluble vitamins

Did you know that some vitamins, such as A, D, E and K, are fat soluble, meaning that without the presence of fat they cannot be absorbed by the body? This means that by simply adding some fats such as nuts, olive oil or avocado to a salad you are giving those vitamins the transporter they need to be absorbed and utilized.

2. Fats for fuel

Fat is the most energy-dense macronutrient of all with 9 kcal per gram but that's not something to fear. It just means that fat is a great source of sustained energy for you to utilize at the right times. Fat also takes longer to digest in the gut so it increases satiety and helps maintain stable blood sugar levels.

3. Healthy hormones

Fat is also necessary for the production of essential hormones. It forms the structural components of healthy cells that are vital for regulating many functions in the body, including the production of sex hormones. This is why extreme low-calorie and low-fat dieting can negatively affect a woman's menstrual cycle.

4. Healthy hair and glowing skin

Often one of the first things my clients notice when increasing their healthy fat intake is the improvement in their skin. If your body lacks the essential omega fatty acids, your skin can appear dry, flaky and dehydrated. Fat builds healthy cell membranes and this helps the body produce the skin's natural oil barrier.

Protein

All proteins are made up of amino acids. Nine of these amino acids are considered essential because the body cannot produce them itself. This means we must include these in the diet. If we don't get enough of these amino acids it can lead to a protein deficiency, which makes it hard for your body to build lean muscle and repair cells. This is why protein forms the basis for my recipes in this book and remains consistent on both training and rest days. If you're vegetarian and there is a recipe you like the look of, simply swap in tofu or Quorn for the meat.

Important functions of protein are:

★ **To build muscle** – every day your body is breaking down proteins, even more so when you train, so it's essential to consume adequate protein in your diet. This allows your body a chance to repair and rebuild lean muscle more quickly.

★ **To regulate metabolism** – every cell requires protein, including your hormones, such as insulin, which is responsible for regulating blood sugar levels.

★ **To ensure healthy cells** – protein is responsible for repairing and maintaining healthy cells found in skin, hair and nails.

Carbohydrates

When it comes to fat loss people often see carbs as the devil and avoid them like the plague, especially after 6pm (what a silly myth that is). This really isn't necessary as it's not carbs that make you gain fat. The body starts to store fat when we consume excess energy. Carbs are actually a great energy source for the muscles to use during intense exercise. That is why in this plan you will utilize more carbohydrates on a training day to fuel your workouts and

> **'PROTEIN FORMS THE BASIS FOR MY RECIPES IN THIS BOOK AND REMAINS CONSISTENT ON BOTH TRAINING AND REST DAYS'**

reduce your carb intake on a rest day, when your body will be gaining the majority of its energy from fats.

Carbohydrates are sugars that come in two main forms: simple and complex, also referred to as simple sugars and starches. The difference between a simple and a complex carb is in how quickly it is digested and absorbed, as well as its structure. Carbohydrates are broken down into glucose by the body and stored in the liver and muscles as glycogen.

Here's a quick lowdown on the types of carbohydrates:

Simple carbs

Simple carbs make things taste sweet and are easily broken down into glucose. Due to their simple structure and quick absorption these types of carbs raise blood glucose levels quickly. Your pancreas releases a hormone called insulin, which works to drive the glucose to the muscles to stabilize blood sugar levels. This insulin response is a good thing after a workout as it shuttles the nutrients from your meal straight into the muscle cells, where they can be used to start the repair and rebuilding process. At other times, though, if your glycogen levels are fully topped up and you continue to take simple carbs on board, your body will start to convert the excess energy and store it as fat.

Simple carbs can be found in things such as fruit, concentrated fruit juice, table sugar, honey, sweets, fizzy drinks, cakes and many packaged cereals. These may provide you with a quick energy boost but what goes up must come down and you will soon feel tired, sluggish and craving more when your blood sugar levels drop.

I call this the sugar monster, and it can be very addictive and difficult to shake off. If you want to stay full of energy my advice is to gradually limit your consumption of these sorts of foods.

Complex carbs

These have a more complex structure and therefore take longer to break down into glucose, meaning that your blood sugar levels don't spike as they do with simple sugars. Instead they can provide you with a steadier supply of energy. They also contain vitamins, minerals and antioxidants.

Good sources include oats, wholegrain rice, quinoa, potatoes, lentils and vegetables. In this plan you will get more of your energy from these sources on training days and less on rest days, when your body will be mainly utilizing fats for energy.

Fibrous carbs

Unlike simple or starchy complex carbs, fibrous carbs, found in vegetables, are not fully digested in the body. These carbs therefore do not elevate blood sugar levels or provide many calories. Essential for gut health, they should ideally be consumed with every meal every day.

Good examples include spinach, broccoli, kale, green beans, cauliflower and courgettes. If you can't stand eating them you could always put them in a shake or smoothie.

How will I be eating?

The recipes in this book are broken down into three different groups:

1. Reduced-carbohydrate meals
2. Carbohydrate-rich meals
3. Snacks and treats

On a training day in this phase you will be consuming three carbohydrate-rich meals and two snacks.

On a rest day you will consume three reduced-carbohydrate meals and two snacks.

You can train at any time of the day and eat your meals and snacks when it suits you. Meal frequency actually has no effect on metabolism, so as long as you consume all of your meals it doesn't matter if you eat them close together or spread out. Just please ignore that myth about not being able to eat carbs in the evening. If you train late your body still needs to be refuelled, so always consume a carb-rich meal post-workout.

The Plan is totally flexible – you can make any of the recipes in this book for breakfast, lunch or dinner. I want you to think outside the cereal box, so if you feel like a burger or burrito for breakfast, go for it!

I've included a few treats in Chapter 5 of this book, but these should be eaten only once or twice a week and only after a workout.

Why eat this way?

On a training day you will be working out at high intensities. During high intensity exercise such as cardio and weight training

> YOU CAN TRAIN AT ANY TIME OF THE DAY AND EAT YOUR MEALS AND SNACKS WHEN IT SUITS YOU

your body will be mainly using carbohydrates for energy, so it's important you fuel your body on these days and also top up your glycogen levels. Remember, glycogen is the stored form of carbohydrates in your body and you do not want to run out if you are training hard.

On rest days you will reduce your carb intake as your body will not be working at high intensity. During low intensity activity such as walking, sitting at your desk and even sleeping, your body utilizes mainly fats for fuel. This is the rationale behind fuelling your body with more carbs on a training day and more fats on a rest day and ensures your body is making use of the correct fuel source at the right time. It works for me and my clients, and will do for you too.

How much should I be eating?

When clients sign up to my online programme, I produce a plan with tailored calories and macros, designed on the basis of responses to a lengthy questionnaire about height, weight, activity levels, age, dieting history and so forth, to guarantee success. With a book like this, I can't match each recipe to each reader, because you all have different energy demands. But I am giving you the template and the basics to create your own successful regime. It is relatively easy to assess whether you need to reduce or increase the portions. I don't want you to think that the portions in this book are necessarily the perfect amount for your body. I want to encourage you to develop your own awareness of your energy intake and output (without relying on complex calorie or macro calculations), and to adjust the meal size accordingly depending on your activity levels and also progress.

My advice is to start with big portions and then see how your body responds. If your body fat isn't melting after 4 weeks, then you can gradually reduce your energy intake to promote fat metabolism. This makes more sense than eating really teeny-weeny portions and cutting calories too low too fast, because if your body stops burning fat you'll have nowhere to go. The key is not to go hungry. Just listen to your body and make small changes if you hit a plateau. Remember, the aim here is to be in a position where your body is still burning fat while you eat as much food as possible. This makes staying lean enjoyable and sustainable.

Listen to your body and make small changes if you hit a plateau

Drink yourself lean

One of the first things I get my clients to consider when trying to get lean and healthy is to increase their water intake. This is because people often overlook the importance of hydration for health and simply don't drink enough.

Being properly hydrated helps support a healthy liver and digestive system. This allows your body to become more efficient at removing toxins, digesting food and metabolizing fat. It will also improve your energy levels, so always aim to maintain a good level of hydration. A reasonable target would be between 2 and 4 litres of water per day. If you really struggle to drink water try adding some fresh lemon or lime for a twist of flavour and avoid drinks that are high in sugar.

Can I booze and lose?

Fun is fun and where there is fun there is often booze. Often the first thing people ask me is, 'Can I still drink alcohol on your plan?' My answer is always the same: 'Yes, sure you can, but the less you booze, the leaner you will get.' This is because alcohol contains 7 kcal of energy per gram – almost as much as fat, which provides 9 kcal per gram. So drinking a few beers or glasses of wine can quickly add up and contribute to your weekly calorie intake, putting your body in a calorie surplus and preventing you from burning fat.

Alcohol is also considered to be 'empty' calories because it provides more energy than it does nutrients. The body cannot store alcohol as it can fat, protein and carbohydrates so it has to get rid of it. This means the body will prioritize burning alcohol over fat or carbohydrates while it's in your system. Boozing puts the brakes on fat-burning and could be the missing link for you between being lean and being 'almost lean'.

Having said this, though, I don't want you to feel like you need to cut alcohol out of your life completely, because that's unrealistic and unnecessary. I certainly don't. Parties, weddings, birthdays, Christmas and work events will always get in your way, so just find a balance and do what it takes to earn the body you want.

GETTING STARTED

2

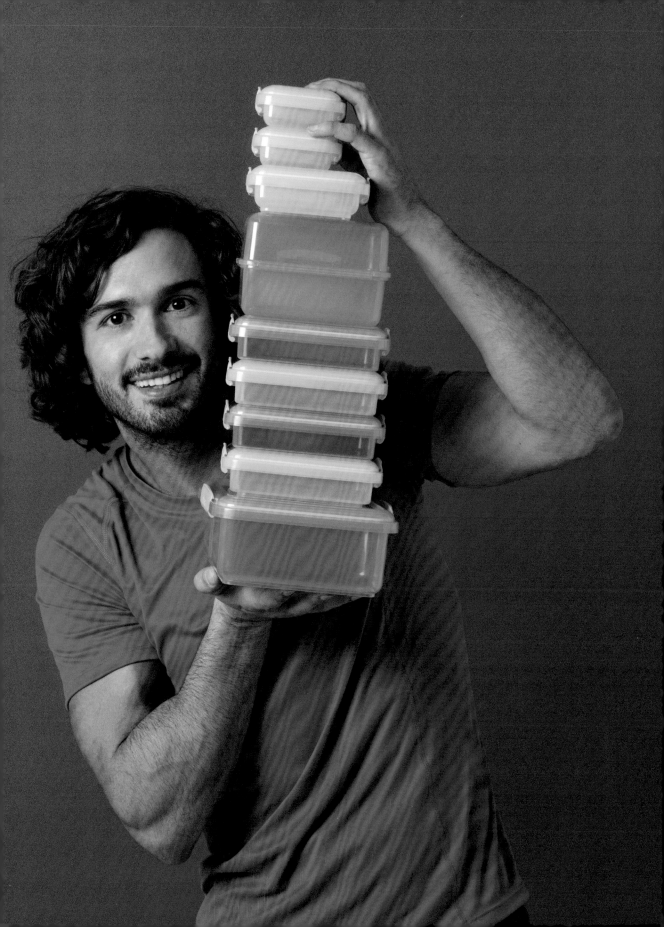

GETTING STARTED

//

PREP LIKE A BOSS

Right, so now you know a bit more about fuelling your body properly it's time to get going. The key to success on the Shape Plan is to be in control of your food intake and this means being able to cook and prepare your meals. I call this 'prepping like a boss'. This may mean prepping your lunch for work the following day or, if you are super-busy, you might prepare meals for the whole week ahead and store them in the fridge or freezer.

The important thing here is to do what works for you and fits into your lifestyle. The less stress the better. There will, of course, be days when you can't prep, or you may forget to take your lunch box into work. It's not the end of the world, but just try your best to prep your meals, avoid eating junk food on the go and keep on track with your goals.

Photos show the real truth of visual progress

TAKE PROGRESS PICS

If you know me, you'll know I'm not a fan of the sad step (bathroom scales), because time and time again I've witnessed it upsetting my clients. Scales are such a poor indicator of progress because they only measure weight. They cannot measure changes in body composition, fitness or confidence so my advice is to DITCH them and take progress pics instead.

The mirror can lie but photos show the real truth of visual progress. I suggest taking front and side-on pics at the end of each month. This will show you real changes over time and motivate you to keep pushing on.

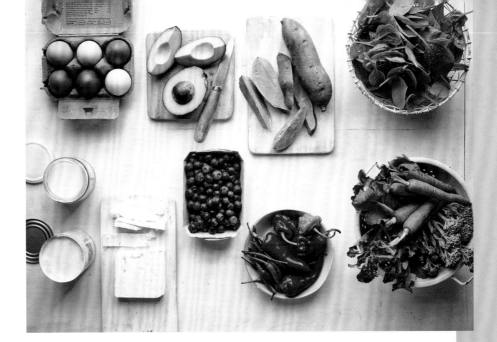

HERO
INGREDIENTS

//

Here's a list of my hero ingredients and why I love them so much:

- Coconut oil – a natural saturated fat perfect for cooking
- **Avocado – the green goddess packed with heart-healthy monounsaturated fat**
- Midget trees – broccoli is packed with important vitamins, and the trees are fun to talk to
- **Coconut milk – perfect for whipping up a curry in a hurry**
- Chillies – dried or fresh, they bring spice to your life
- **Eggs – the home of healthy fats and good any time of the day**
- Spinach – Popeye used it to get strong and so do I
- **Feta cheese – because it tastes unreal on almost anything at any time**
- Blueberries – I love them on my pancakes or oats and they are full of antioxidants
- **Sweet potatoes – because I love making mash, fries and fritters**

	MONDAY	TUESDAY	WEDNESDAY	THURSDAY	FRIDAY	SATURDAY	SUNDAY
Training am		Arms	Rest day		Rest day	Shoulders	Rest day
Post-workout		Joe's protein shake				Joe's protein shake	
Meal 1	Overnight oats	Protein pancakes	Salmon and feta frittata	Protein pancakes	Chunky monkey smoothie	Cinnamon French toast	Grilled salmon with avocado
Snack	30g nuts	Walnut whip hummus	Veg patch juice	75g blueberries	2 energy balls	30g nuts	Roasted midget trees with tahini
Meal 2	Korean pork-fried rice	Fully loaded chicken pitta	Grilled sea bass with minted peas	Prawn and chilli tagliatelle	Terry the tuna with melon and feta	Pesto penne with grilled tuna	Pork chop, feta and beetroot
Snack	Boiled egg	Apple	85g beef jerky	2 energy balls	30g nuts	Apple	Boiled egg
Training pm	Chest and back			Legs			
Post-workout	Joe's protein shake			Joe's protein shake			
Meal 3	Aussie bum burger	Monkfish kebabs with tabbouleh	Philly cheese and jalapeño steak	Hot and sour beef noodles	Chipotle lamb and tomatoes with spinach	Hot and sour beef noodles	Chicken rendang

My Shape Plan
perfect week

• • • • • • • • • • • • • • • •

I've created this table to show you a typical week for me, using the recipes and the workouts in this book. Hopefully it will give you some ideas to plan your own week. Use the table opposite to help you prep like a boss.

	MONDAY	TUESDAY	WEDNESDAY	THURSDAY	FRIDAY	SATURDAY	SUNDAY
Training am							
Post-workout							
Meal 1							
Snack							
Meal 2							
Snack							
Training pm							
Post-workout							
Meal 3							

USE THIS TABLE TO PLAN YOUR OWN MEALS AND WORKOUTS FOR THE WEEK

Don't give up

. . . .

Over the past two years I have helped hundreds of thousands of people overcome poor lifelong eating habits to take control and get in shape. One thing I have come to learn is how challenging it can be for people to change. Many people have strong emotional connections with food, which can lead to undereating, overeating or bingeing. The important thing to remember is that you're not alone and that you are human. We all have good and bad days when it comes to eating. You may not win every day but as long as you refocus and don't let a bad day of eating ruin your week you will still make progress.

REDUCED-CARBOHYDRATE RECIPES

3

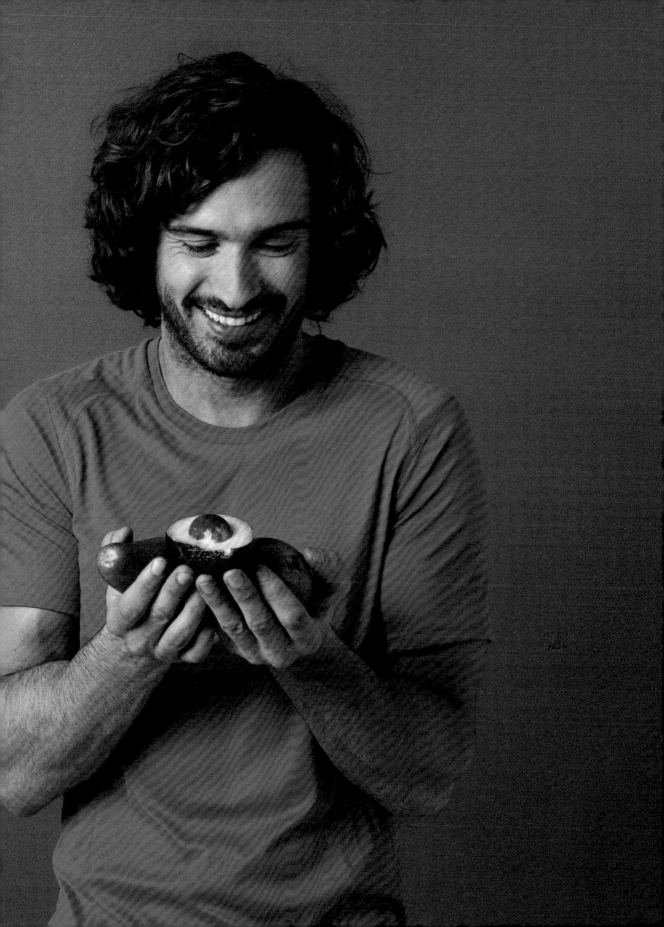

CHUNKY MONKEY SMOOTHIE

SERVES 1

This cheeky monkey is perfect for peanut butter lovers on the move. It almost tastes like a Snickers bar too . . . Ooooh guilty!

REDUCED-CARB INGREDIENTS

½ banana, peeled and roughly chopped
½ tbsp cacao powder
1½ tbsp peanut butter
250ml almond milk
1 scoop (30g) chocolate protein powder
2 tsp sesame seeds

METHOD

Chuck all of the ingredients into a blender and whizz up until you reach a roughly smooth drink.

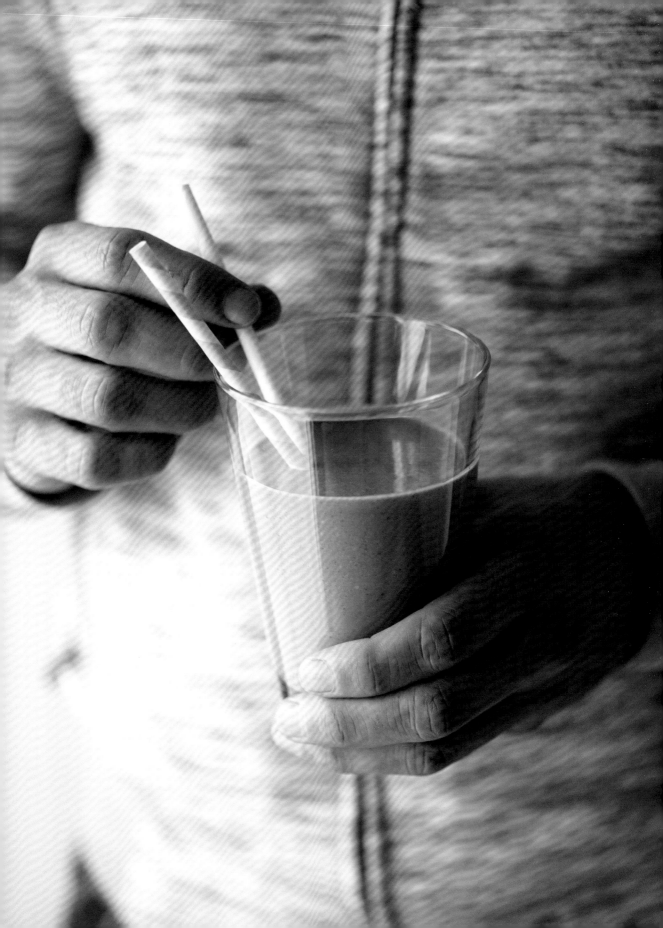

REDUCED-CARB
INGREDIENTS

2 rashers of smoked back
  bacon
2 eggs
1 avocado, de-stoned and
  peeled
¼ red pepper, de-seeded and
  finely chopped
1 tsp sesame oil
juice of 1 lime
1 spring onion, trimmed and
  finely sliced
salt and pepper
2 crispbreads (I like to use
  Original Ryvita)
1 tbsp coriander leaves
½ red chilli, finely chopped –
  optional

SMASHED AVOCADO WITH KEVIN BACON

Three of my favourite things all on one plate: avocado,
egg and bacon? Yes, please #FatsMeUp. I'm all about that
crispy bacon under the grill, too.

METHOD

Bring a saucepan of water to the boil and preheat your grill
to maximum.

Place the bacon rashers on the grill pan or a baking tray and
cook under the grill for 3 minutes on each side. Carefully
lower the eggs into the boiling water and boil for 6 minutes.
When the time is up, pour the hot water out of the pan and
fill back up with cold water.

While the bacon and eggs are cooking, put the avocado flesh,
red pepper, sesame oil, lime juice and spring onion in a bowl
along with a generous pinch of salt and pepper. Using the
back of a fork, crush and mix the ingredients together until
they are well combined.

Drain the excess fat from the cooked bacon on a piece of
clean kitchen roll.

Lay the crispbreads on your plate, top with the bacon and then
dollop on the smashed avocado. Peel the eggs and sit them
proudly on top or alongside, scatter the whole lot with fresh
coriander and chopped chilli, if using, and get stuck in.

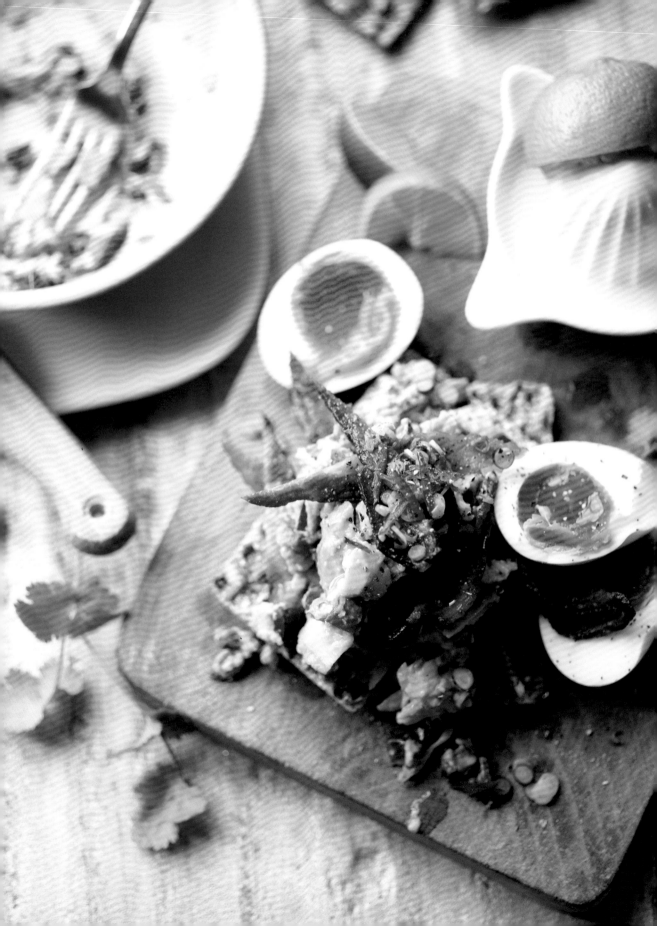

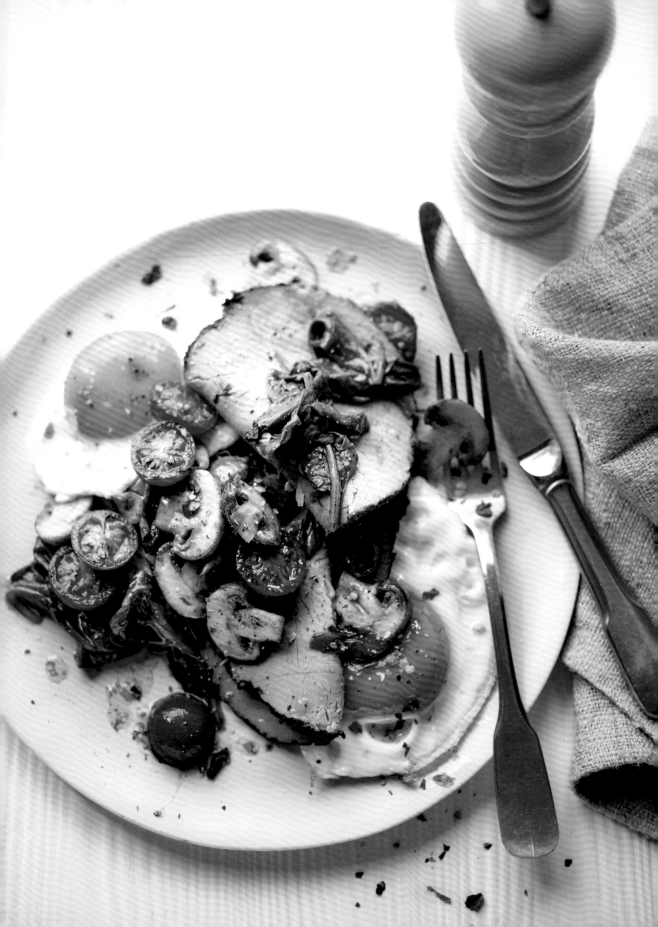

GREENS, EGGS AND HAM

SERVES 1

REDUCED-CARB
INGREDIENTS

½ tbsp butter
4 chestnut mushrooms,
  sliced
4 cherry tomatoes, halved
salt and pepper
large handful of baby spinach
  leaves
2 eggs
2 thick slices of unsmoked
  deli-style ham (about 240g)
dried chilli flakes – if you like
  a bit of heat

Ditch the sugary cereals once and for all. They don't provide you with 'sustained energy' like the adverts say. It's all lies and marketing. This breakfast is high in protein and healthy fats and is exactly what your body needs. Don't get that nasty cheap re-formed meat, though . . . head to the deli counter for the real stuff.

METHOD

Preheat your grill to maximum.

Heat the butter in a frying pan over a medium to high heat. When hot and bubbling, chuck in the mushrooms and tomatoes. Fry the ingredients for 2 minutes, stirring every now and then – it's nice to let the mushrooms colour a little. Season with salt and pepper.

Add the spinach to the pan and toss with the mushrooms and tomatoes until wilted. Reduce the heat to medium to low, arrange the ingredients into a pile and move them to one side of the pan. Crack the eggs into the other side of the pan and let them fry on the base for 1 minute.

When you are happy the eggs have cooked on the bottom, slide the whole pan under the grill and cook for about 1–2 minutes depending on how well cooked you like your eggs.

When ready to eat, place your ham slices onto a plate with the mushroom and egg mix – sprinkle artistically with a few chilli flakes to give your day a proper kick-start.

SALMON AND FETA FRITTATA . . . BOSH!

SERVES 1

MAKE AHEAD

INGREDIENTS

3 eggs
40g smoked salmon, thinly
  sliced
1 red chilli, roughly chopped
  – remove the seeds if you
  don't like it hot
1 tbsp chopped chives
40g feta, drained
black pepper
½ tbsp coconut oil
handful of baby spinach
  leaves
handful of rocket, to serve

You can't beat a fatty frittata for breakfast. This one's got the lot: omega-3s from the salmon, monounsaturated fats from the eggs and saturated fats from the coconut oil and cheese. If you don't like salmon you could always use some good quality ham or turkey bacon instead.

METHOD

Preheat your grill to maximum.

Crack the eggs into a bowl, add the smoked salmon, chilli and chives and crumble in the feta. Season with a generous pinch of black pepper, but no salt.

Melt the coconut oil in a small, non-stick frying pan over a medium to high heat. Drop in the spinach and stir until wilted. Pour the egg mixture into the pan and move the eggs around, drawing in the cooked edges and manoeuvring the raw egg into the gaps. When all the egg is semi-cooked, leave to fry, without stirring, for 1 minute.

After 1 minute, slide the frying pan under the grill and cook until the top of the frittata is bubbling. Remove the pan from under the heat (be careful as the handle may be hot). Slide the frittata onto a plate and top with the rocket.

INDIAN OMELETTE

SERVES 1

Spice up your morning with this delicious Indian-inspired omelette. You might think I'm mad throwing these sorts of spices about at breakfast but trust me, it's the perfect fuel to set you up for the day and tastes wicked.

REDUCED-CARB INGREDIENTS

½ tbsp coconut oil
½ small red onion, finely diced
1 green chilli, de-seeded and finely sliced
1 tbsp chopped coriander, plus a little extra for serving
3 eggs
pinch of turmeric
black pepper
½ tsp garam masala
175g cooked skinless chicken breast, roughly shredded
15g toasted cashews, roughly chopped

METHOD

Melt the coconut oil in a small, non-stick frying pan over a medium heat. Add the onion, chilli and chopped coriander and fry for 2 minutes.

While the ingredients are cooking away, crack the eggs into a bowl and add the turmeric along with a pinch of black pepper. Whisk up the eggs and spice until they are well combined.

When the onions have had their 2 minutes, sprinkle in the garam masala and fry, stirring almost constantly, for 30 seconds. Increase the heat to medium to high and pour in the egg mixture. Fry the egg, drawing in the cooked egg from the sides, for about 30 seconds, or until it resembles scrambled egg. Spread the egg across the base of the pan to allow it to brown.

Scatter the cooked chicken over the middle of the omelette and, when you are happy the eggs are cooked enough to hold their shape, turn off the heat and fold one half of the omelette over the chicken.

Transfer the omelette to a plate and top with the chopped cashews and a final sprinkling of chopped coriander.

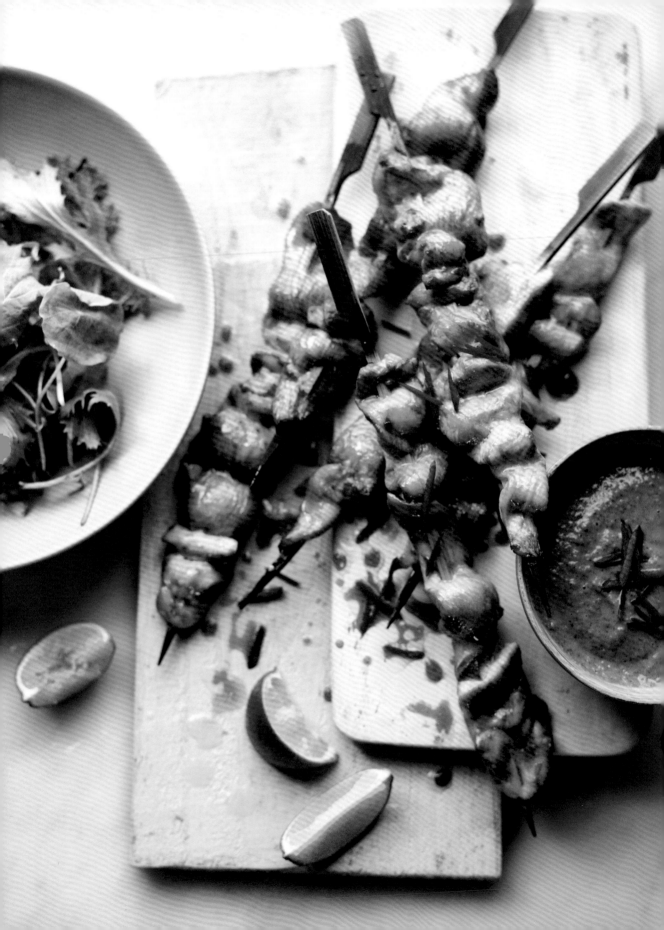

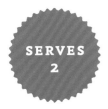

REDUCED-CARB
MAKE AHEAD
INGREDIENTS

3 cloves garlic
2 x 240g skinless chicken
  breast fillets, sliced into long
  1cm thick strips
3 tbsp light soy sauce
1 lemongrass stalk, tender
  white part only, finely sliced
1½ tbsp fish sauce
2cm ginger, finely chopped
1 red chilli, roughly chopped –
  remove the seeds if you
  don't like it hot
2 tbsp natural peanut butter –
  crunchy or smooth, it's up
  to you
4 spring onions
2 tsp of honey
sprigs of coriander, to serve –
  optional
lime wedges, to serve

★ Serve with a fresh green
salad.

CHICKEN SATAY SKEWERS

This is one of my favourite things to make for a dinner party starter but it's also perfect for a low-carb lunch boxed up and taken to work with a green salad. If you don't have skewers, don't worry, just lay your chicken strips out on a baking tray.

METHOD

Preheat your grill to maximum.

Finely chop one of the garlic cloves. Place the chicken strips in a bowl and add the chopped garlic and 1 tablespoon of the light soy sauce. Mix the ingredients together. Thread the chicken onto skewers, making sure not to pack them too tightly otherwise they won't cook. Place the skewered chicken on the grill pan or a baking tray and slide under the grill. Cook the chicken for about 5 minutes on each side or until it is fully cooked through. Check by slicing into one of the larger pieces to make sure the meat is white all the way through, with no raw pink bits left.

While the chicken is cooking, place the remaining garlic cloves and soy sauce in a blender along with the lemongrass, fish sauce, ginger, chilli, peanut butter, spring onions, a little drizzle of honey and a splash of warm water. Blitz until just smooth.

Serve up your chicken skewers smothered in the delicious satay sauce, topped with coriander sprigs, if using, and with lime wedges to squeeze over.

★ TOP TIP

Here's a little tip for you. Soak your wooden skewers in cold water for 10 minutes before you load up the chicken and stick them under the grill. This stops the wood from burning and you having a fire on your hands!

GRILLED SALMON WITH AVOCADO, FETA AND PUMPKIN SEEDS

SERVES 1

REDUCED-CARB

INGREDIENTS

drizzle of olive oil
1 x 240g salmon fillet, skin on
2 tbsp pumpkin seeds
salt
1 avocado, peeled, de-stoned
  and roughly chopped
¼ red onion, finely chopped
2 tsp sesame oil
1 tbsp chopped coriander
40g feta, drained
handful of watercress, to serve
juice of 1 lime, to serve –
  optional

Wow, talk about healthy fats . . . this one not only looks and tastes great but is also literally rammed with goodness.

METHOD

Preheat your grill to maximum.

Drizzle a little olive oil over the skin side of the salmon, place on the grill pan or a baking tray and slide under the hot grill. Cook for 6 minutes on the skin side, before carefully flipping and grilling for a further 4 minutes. Turn the grill off and leave the salmon to keep warm until you're ready to eat.

While the salmon is cooking, tip the pumpkin seeds into a dry frying pan and toast over a high heat for about 2 minutes, or until they start turning brown and popping. Season with a little salt and leave in the pan.

Using the back of a fork, break up the avocado in a bowl. Add the onion, sesame oil and coriander. Mix the whole lot together until the ingredients are well combined.

Slide your salmon onto a plate, removing the skin as you go. Pile up the guacamole, slice and scatter over the feta, and finish with a sprinkling of toasted pumpkin seeds, a pile of watercress and a squeeze of lime juice, if using.

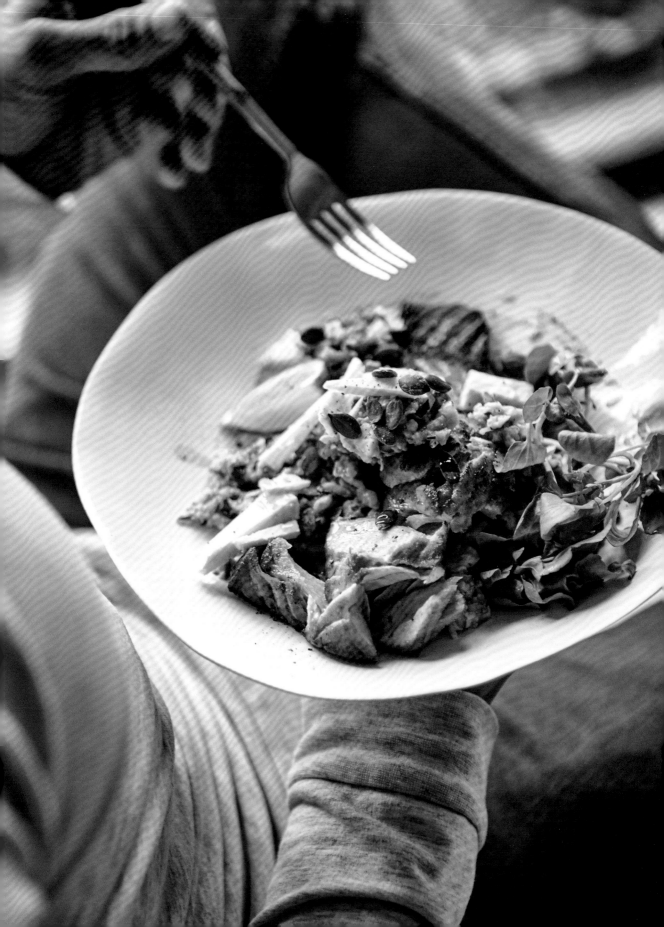

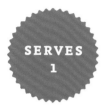

PHILLY CHEESE AND JALAPEÑO STEAK

Oh, wow, sirloin steak with two types of melted cheese? Sorry, this doesn't need an introduction, it needs an award – the tastiest meal of the week goes to . . .

REDUCED-CARB INGREDIENTS

½ tbsp coconut oil

1 x 300g sirloin steak at room temperature, trimmed of visible fat

salt and pepper

½ red onion, sliced into 6 thin wedges

3 chestnut mushrooms, finely sliced

2 large handfuls of spinach leaves

2 thick slices of mozzarella

1 thick slice of mature cheddar

1 red chilli, finely sliced – remove the seeds if you don't like it hot

6 jarred jalapeño slices – more if you like it hot

METHOD

Melt the coconut oil in a frying pan over a high heat. Season the steak with salt and pepper before laying gently in the pan. Fry the steak for 2 minutes on each side, then remove to a plate.

Reduce the heat to medium to high and add the onion and mushrooms. Stir-fry the ingredients for 2 minutes until just softened. Mix in half the spinach and let it wilt.

Take the pan off the heat and push the vegetables to one side. Lay the steak back in the pan and pile the vegetables on top. Place the cheese slices over the vegetables, put the pan back on the hob and put a lid on the pan (if you don't have a lid then just cover with a plate).

Cook the steak like this for a further minute, by which time the cheese should have melted. Slide the steak from the pan onto a plate, scatter with chilli and jalapeño slices and serve with the remaining spinach leaves.

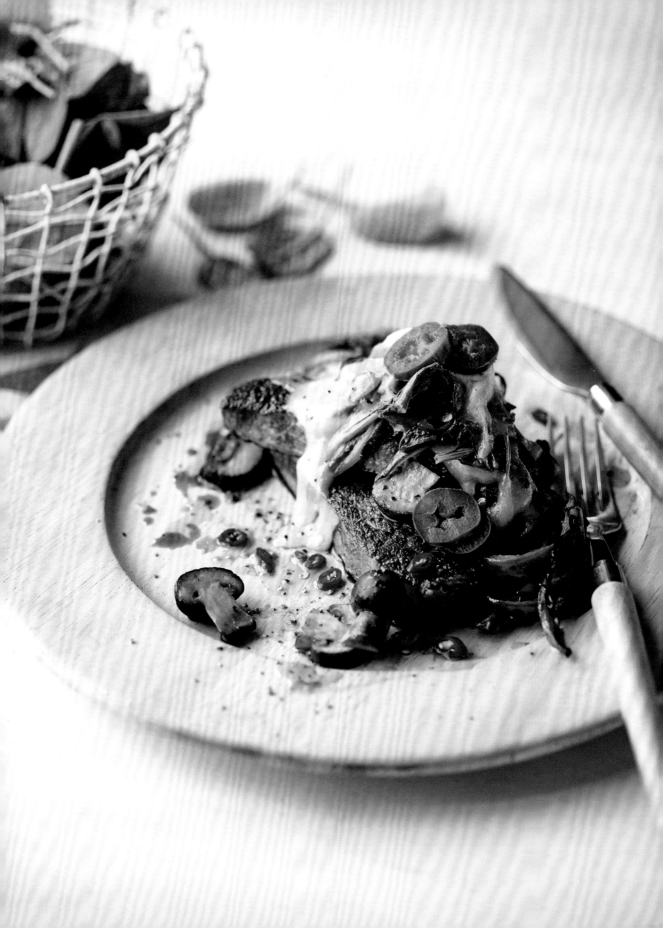

CHICKEN BREAST WITH HERBY CREAM SAUCE

SERVES 1

REDUCED-CARB
INGREDIENTS

½ tbsp coconut oil
¼ leek, washed, trimmed and
  finely sliced
1 clove garlic, finely chopped
1 x 240g skinless chicken
  breast fillet, sliced into 1cm
  thick strips
1½ tbsp mascarpone
salt and pepper
1 tbsp chopped chives
½ tbsp chopped tarragon
1 tbsp chopped parsley
2 large handfuls of baby
  spinach leaves
juice of 1 lemon, to serve

There's nothing worse than eating bland, boring, bone-dry chicken breast all the time. This absolute creamer is here to the rescue. The sauce is well naughty and once you cream up there's no going back.

METHOD

Melt the coconut oil in a wok or large frying pan over a medium to high heat. Chuck in the leek and garlic and stir-fry for 1 minute until softened.

Add the chicken strips to the pan and continue to stir-fry for 2–3 minutes, by which time the chicken should be lightly coloured and cooked through. Check by slicing into one of the larger pieces to make sure the meat is white all the way through, with no raw pink bits left.

Reduce the heat to medium and dollop in the mascarpone followed swiftly by 2 tablespoons of water and a generous pinch of salt and pepper. Gently stir the ingredients until the mascarpone has melted into the liquid and created a creamy sauce.

Add in all the chopped herbs and the spinach. Gently stir the spinach into the rest of the ingredients until it has fully wilted. Taste and season again with a little salt and pepper if you feel it is needed.

Serve up with a squeeze of fresh lemon. Yum.

SERVES 1

REDUCED-CARB INGREDIENTS

1 x 180g skinless salmon fillet, chopped into 2cm chunks
6 raw prawns, peeled
juice of 1 lime
salt and pepper
½ tbsp coconut oil
1 star anise
4 spring onions, finely sliced
2 cloves garlic, chopped
2cm ginger, chopped
1 large red chilli, split down the middle
1 lemongrass stalk, tender white part only, finely chopped
1 tsp turmeric
4 baby sweetcorn, sliced lengthways
30g mange tout
½ x 200ml tin of coconut milk
1 tbsp fish sauce
chopped coriander, to serve

PRAWN AND SALMON LAKSA

This is another one of my favourite curry dishes and so easy to prepare. If you don't like prawns or salmon you could do the same recipe with chicken.

METHOD

Place the salmon and prawns in a bowl, squeeze over the lime juice and sprinkle with a little salt and pepper. Leave the seafood to marinate while you carry on.

Melt the coconut oil in a wok or large frying pan over a medium to high heat. Throw in the star anise, spring onions, garlic, ginger, chilli and lemongrass. Stir-fry the ingredients for 2 minutes. Add the turmeric, baby sweetcorn and mange tout and continue to stir-fry for a further minute.

Pour in the coconut milk and stir to combine with the rest of the ingredients. Bring the liquid to the boil and simmer for 1 minute. Drop in the marinated salmon and prawns, bring the liquid back up to the boil and simmer for 30 seconds, until the fish is cooked through and the prawns are pink.

Remove the laksa from the heat and stir through the fish sauce and chopped coriander.

HOLY MONKFISH

SERVES 1

'How can he possibly make a stew in 15 minutes?' I hear you ask. Just because it's called a stew doesn't mean we have to sit around for hours waiting for it to cook, does it? The flavours are still there and the monkfish cooks super-quick, so 15 minutes is very doable . . . Enjoy!

REDUCED-CARB INGREDIENTS

1 tbsp coconut oil

½ red onion, finely diced

½ courgette, trimmed and diced

¼ aubergine, trimmed and diced

1 clove garlic, roughly chopped

2 tsp smoked paprika

2 tsp tomato puree

1 x 200g fillet of monkfish, trimmed and chopped into chunks

50g tinned kidney beans, drained and rinsed

2 tbsp ground almonds

2 tbsp chopped parsley, to serve – optional

★ Serve with a big portion of your favourite greens such as spinach, kale, broccoli, mange tout or green beans.

METHOD

Melt the coconut oil in a wok or large frying pan over a medium to high heat. Chuck in the onion, courgette, aubergine and garlic. Fry, stirring regularly, for 4–5 minutes until the vegetables are just softening.

Sprinkle in the smoked paprika and add the tomato puree, the chunks of monkfish and the kidney beans. Continue to stir-fry for 1 minute before pouring in 150ml water.

Bring the liquid to the boil and simmer for 2 minutes, or until you are sure the fish is cooked through. This can be tested by pulling out one of the thickest pieces and cutting it in half to make sure it has turned from raw, pale flesh to cooked bright white.

When you are happy that the fish is cooked through, turn off the heat and stir in the ground almonds and chopped parsley, if using.

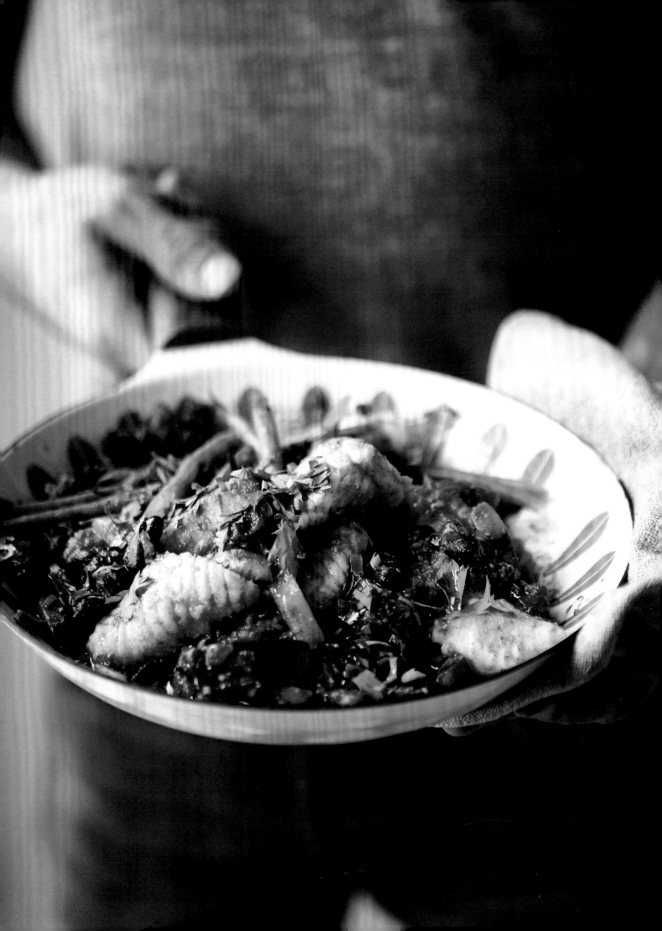

PORK CHOP, FETA AND BEETROOT

I'm not sure why but beetroot and feta just go so well together. If you don't like pork you could use a chicken breast here instead.

REDUCED-CARB INGREDIENTS

1 large pork chop – roughly 275g with most fat removed
salt and pepper
1 cooked beetroot, roughly sliced into 6 wedges
1 tbsp balsamic or red wine vinegar
1 tbsp chopped toasted hazelnuts
1 tbsp olive oil
1 spring onion, finely sliced
30g feta
½ avocado, de-stoned, peeled and sliced into wedges
handful of baby spinach leaves

METHOD

Preheat your grill to maximum.

Place the pork chop on the grill pan, season generously with salt and pepper and slide under the grill. Cook for 7 minutes, flip and then cook for a further 4 minutes before turning off the grill and leaving the chop to rest for 1 minute. Check it's cooked through by cutting into one of the thicker parts to make sure there is no pink left.

Meanwhile, place the beetroot, vinegar, hazelnuts, olive oil and spring onion in a bowl. Season the ingredients with salt and pepper and toss to mix.

Place your cooked pork chop on a plate, pile up the beetroot salad, crumble the feta all over and serve with the avocado wedges and some baby spinach leaves.

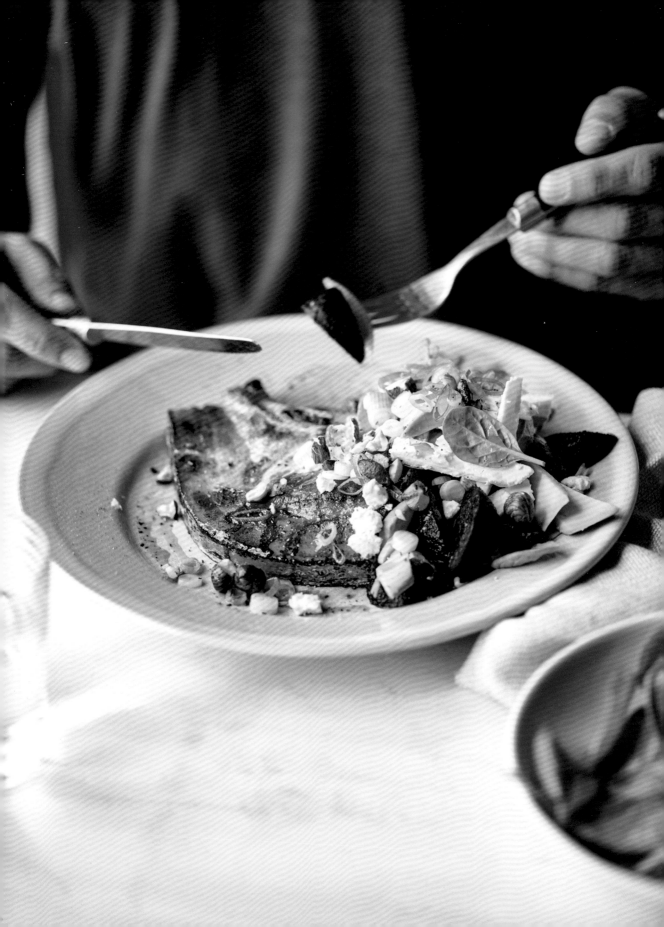

SPICY SCRAMBLED EGGS WITH CHORIZO

REDUCED-CARB INGREDIENTS

½ tbsp coconut oil

75g cooking chorizo, diced into 1cm pieces

¼ courgette, diced into 1cm pieces

50g kale, stalks removed and leaves roughly chopped into small pieces

2 spring onions, finely sliced

1 red chilli, finely sliced – remove the seeds if you don't like it hot

¼ red pepper, de-seeded and finely sliced

3 eggs

black pepper

chopped coriander, to serve

I'm a massive fan of eating fats and this meal with eggs and chorizo cooked in coconut oil is perfect. It will give you all the energy you need to go out and win.

METHOD

Melt the coconut oil in a wok or large frying pan over a medium to high heat. Add the chorizo and stir-fry for 2 minutes.

Now add the courgette, kale, spring onions, chilli and red pepper. Stir-fry for 2–3 minutes until the ingredients start to brown. Pour in 2 tablespoons of water, letting it steam up and disappear – this will help ensure all the ingredients are cooked through.

Whisk together the eggs, adding a generous pinch of pepper to the mix. Pour the eggs into the pan with the rest of the ingredients and cook them as you would scrambled eggs – drawing the cooked egg from the edges into the middle, until the egg is all cooked. I like to let the bottom brown a little.

Slide the bulked-up scrambled eggs onto a plate and scatter over the chopped coriander.

SAMMY THE SEA BASS WITH SALSA VERDE

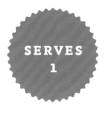

Salsa verde is just a fancy name for a load of herbs mixed together – it works so well with the crispy skin of the grilled sea bass.

REDUCED-CARB INGREDIENTS

2 x 125g sea bass fillets,
  skin on
2 tbsp olive oil, plus a little
  to drizzle
salt and pepper
1 tbsp sherry, balsamic or red
  wine vinegar
1 tbsp finely chopped dill
1 tbsp finely chopped chives
1 tbsp finely chopped basil
1 tbsp finely chopped parsley
¼ red onion, finely diced
1 ripe avocado
½ red pepper, roughly
  chopped into 1cm pieces
30g walnuts, roughly chopped
juice of 1 lime, to serve

METHOD

Preheat your grill to maximum.

Lay the bass fillets on a baking tray lined with baking parchment. Drizzle with a little of the olive oil and sprinkle with salt. Grill the fish close to the element for 7–8 minutes without turning. Turn off the heat and leave until you are ready to serve.

While the fish is cooking, pour 2 tablespoons of the olive oil into a bowl and add your chosen vinegar, the dill, chives, basil, parsley and onion. Mix the ingredients together thoroughly.

Cut your avocado in half, remove the stone and scoop out big chunks of the flesh, using a spoon. Place in a bowl and add the red pepper, walnuts and a generous pinch of salt and pepper.

Serve the grilled sea bass with the avocado mix, topped with the salsa verde and a generous squeeze of lime juice.

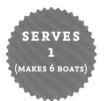

REDUCED-CARB
MAKE AHEAD
INGREDIENTS

30g mayonnaise
70g fat-free Greek yoghurt
2 tsp tomato puree
2 spring onions, finely sliced
1 tbsp curry powder
juice of 1 lemon
salt and pepper
250g cooked skinless chicken
  breast, sliced into 1–2cm
  pieces
1 baby gem lettuce, leaves
  separated
½ avocado, de-stoned, peeled
  and sliced lengthways into
  thin wedges
½ mango, de-stoned, peeled
  and sliced lengthways into
  thin wedges
chopped coriander, to serve –
  optional
flaked almonds, to serve –
  optional

CURRY CHICKEN LETTUCE BOATS

This one makes a great starter if you've got some friends coming over. If you're not into the whole 'boat' thing, just pair the chicken with a nice big salad.

METHOD

Place the mayo, yoghurt, tomato puree, spring onions, curry powder and lemon juice in a bowl along with a generous pinch of salt and pepper. Mix the ingredients together until they become a smooth sauce.

Fold the chicken pieces through the sauce. Lay out 6 of the biggest lettuce leaves and divide the chicken mixture equally among the 'boats'.

Top each boat with a few slices of avocado and mango and finish with a sprinkling of chopped coriander (if using). Gracefully attack your boats with a knife and fork, or alternatively stuff them into your mouth.

★ TOP TIP

Homemade mayo is a joy and pretty easy to make if you have a food processor. Go light with mayo as it is high in fat – even for the reduced-carb meals try not to exceed 30g or so of mayo. Because of the raw egg, pregnant women should give this a miss.

Makes about 200ml

1 egg yolk
¼ tsp Dijon mustard
1 tsp white wine vinegar
130ml vegetable oil

Place all the ingredients into a blender and blitz until smooth and thick. Use straight away or store in an airtight container in the fridge.

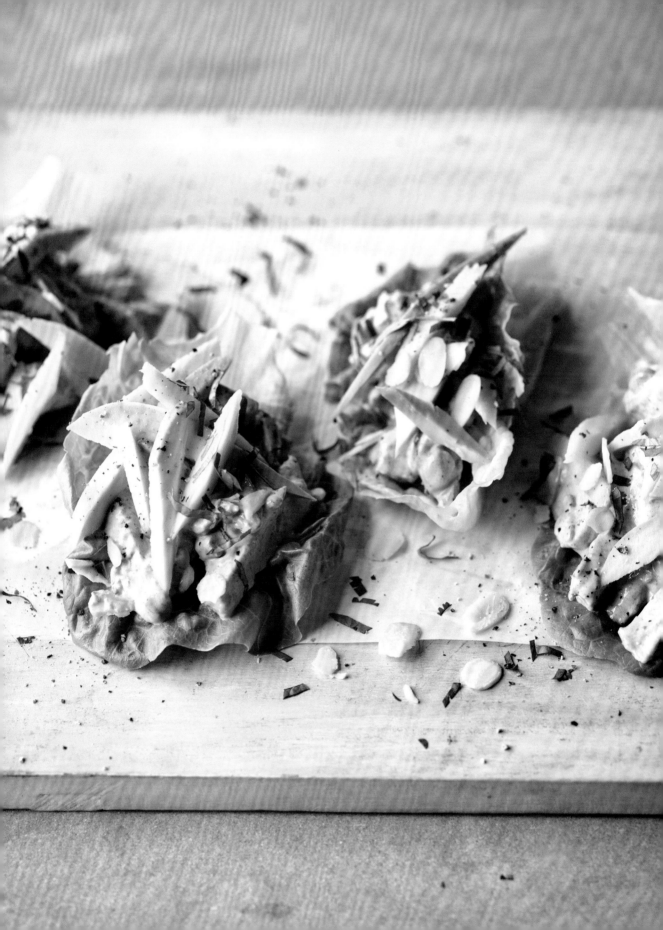

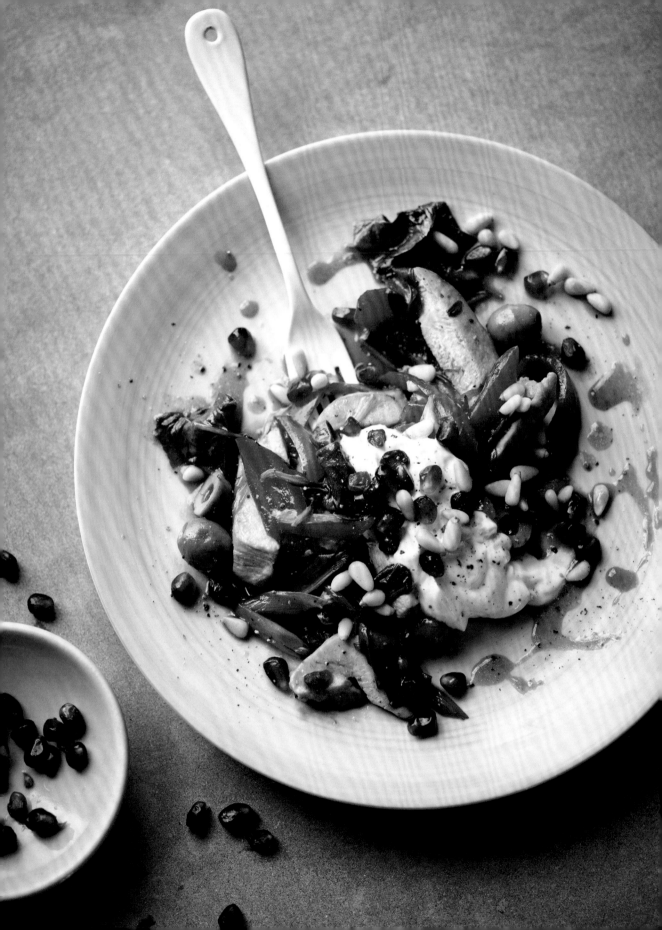

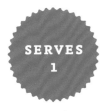

REDUCED-CARB INGREDIENTS

¼ chicken stock cube
small pinch of saffron strands
1 tbsp coconut oil
½ red pepper, de-seeded and
  sliced into 1cm strips
3 spring onions, sliced into
  2cm long pieces
1 x 240g skinless chicken
  breast fillet, sliced into
  6 pieces
salt and pepper
½ preserved lemon, roughly
  chopped
5 pitted green olives
2 large handfuls of baby
  spinach leaves
1 tbsp full-fat Greek yoghurt
20g pine nuts
1 tbsp pomegranate seeds
chopped parsley, to serve –
  optional

MY BIG FAT GREEK CHICKEN

I was a bit unsure about preserved lemons when I first found them but they are so full of flavour and, when combined with olives, they really bring this dish to life. You can find them in most supermarkets.

METHOD

Put the kettle on to boil. Crumble the stock cube into a jug and drop in the saffron strands. Pour over 100ml of boiling water and stir the ingredients together. Leave to infuse while you crack on with the rest of the recipe.

Melt the coconut oil in a large frying pan over a medium to high heat. Add the red pepper, spring onions and chicken breast pieces along with a sprinkle of salt and pepper. Fry the ingredients, stirring occasionally, for 2 minutes.

Increase the heat to maximum, drop in the preserved lemon and green olives and then pour in the infused chicken stock. Bring the whole lot to the boil and simmer for 2–3 minutes, or until you are sure the chicken is cooked through. Check by slicing into one of the thickest pieces to make sure the meat is white all the way through, with no raw pink bits left.

When you are happy the chicken is fully cooked, remove the pan from the heat and stir through the spinach – the residual heat will wilt the leaves.

Serve up the chicken topped with the yoghurt, pine nuts, pomegranate seeds and some chopped parsley, if using.

TERRY THE TUNA WITH MELON AND FETA

REDUCED-CARB
MAKE AHEAD

INGREDIENTS

1 x 250g tuna steak
drizzle of olive oil
salt and pepper
10 large chunks of
   watermelon (about 200g)
75g feta, crumbled
25g walnuts, roughly chopped
2 tbsp olive oil
1 tsp nigella seeds (black
   onion seeds)
handful of baby spinach
   leaves
handful of basil leaves

This is one of those really healthy super-fresh-tasting meals that you know is good for your insides. You can box this one up and take it to work for lunch or have it at home any day of the week.

METHOD

Start by preheating a griddle pan.

Rub the tuna steak with olive oil, making sure the whole steak has a light sheen of oil. Season with salt and pepper, and when the griddle pan is hot, place the fish on it. Griddle the tuna for about 90 seconds on each side before removing and leaving to rest.

To make the salad, chuck the watermelon chunks in a bowl and add the feta, walnuts, olive oil, nigella seeds, spinach and basil leaves and gently stir to mix the ingredients. Grind in some fresh pepper, and a little salt if you think it needs it.

Serve up the tuna steak with the fresh salad.

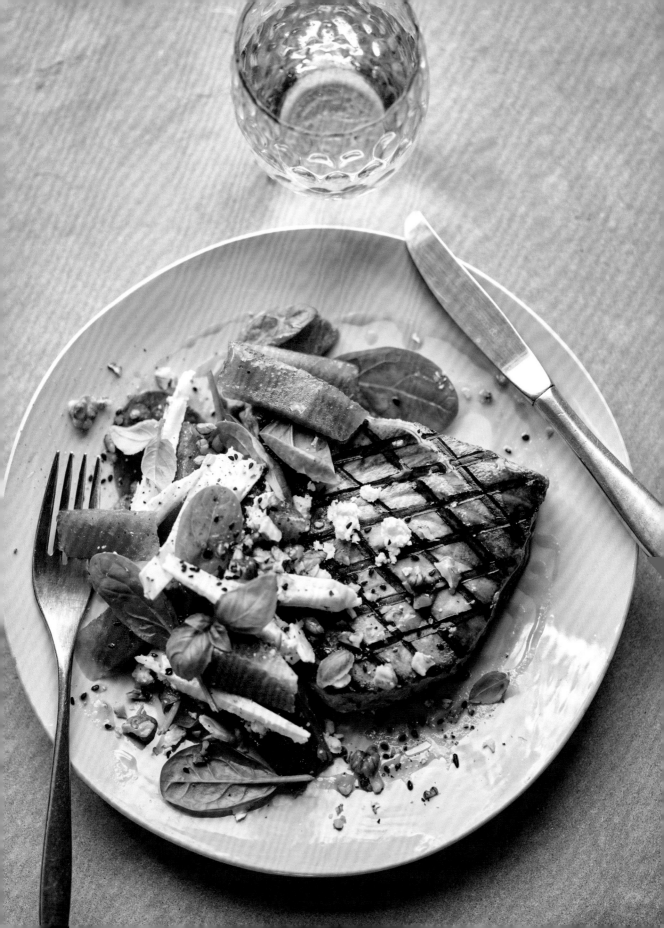

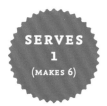

REDUCED-CARB
MAKE AHEAD
GOOD TO FREEZE
INGREDIENTS

1 x 250g cod fillet, skinned and
  roughly chopped
1 red chilli, roughly chopped –
  remove the seeds if you don't
  like it hot
1 lemongrass stalk, tender
  white part only, roughly
  chopped
2 spring onions, roughly
  chopped
2 tbsp roughly chopped
  coriander
1½ tbsp fish sauce
1 egg
2 tbsp desiccated coconut
1 tbsp coconut oil
1 tbsp rice wine vinegar
1 tsp toasted sesame oil
¼ cucumber, sliced into 1cm
  half-moons
2 tbsp salted peanuts, roughly
  chopped
juice of 1 lime, to serve

★ Serve with a big fresh salad
or a pile of felled midget
trees (tender-stem broccoli)
and spinach or green beans.

TASTY THAI FISH CAKES

If you like a bit of Thai food then this recipe will be right up
your street. Ready in minutes, it's easy to batch-cook and
freeze afterwards. Just lay the fish cakes on a lined baking tray
and freeze. Once frozen, they can be stacked up in containers
and when you're ready to eat, heat them in a pan or oven.

METHOD

Chuck the cod, chilli, lemongrass, spring onions, coriander,
1 tablespoon of the fish sauce, egg and coconut into a
food processor. Pulse the ingredients until they are well
combined and are just short of becoming a paste.

With damp hands, shape the mix into six balls and give
them a little pat to flatten them slightly into roughly the
shape of a small ice hockey puck.

Melt the coconut oil in a large frying pan over a medium to
high heat. Lay the fish cakes in the pan and fry them for about
3 minutes on each side, or until they are fully cooked through.
To ensure they are cooked, break one open and check that the
flesh has turned from a raw pale colour to cooked bright white.

While the fish cakes are cooking, mix together the rice wine
vinegar, the remaining ½ tablespoon of fish sauce and the
sesame oil. Pour the dressing over the cucumber half-moons
and toss to coat the pieces.

Drain the cooked fish cakes on a piece of kitchen roll and
serve with the dressed cucumber, a generous sprinkling of
chopped peanuts and a squeeze of lime juice.

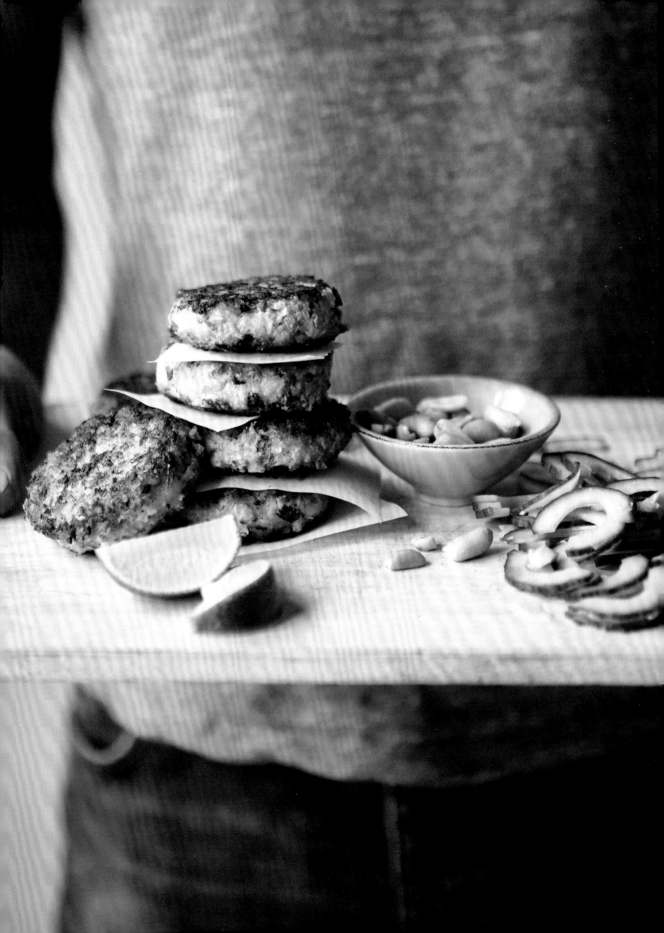

REDUCED-CARB
MAKE AHEAD
GOOD TO FREEZE
INGREDIENTS

1 tbsp coconut oil
5 spring onions, finely sliced
1 lemongrass stalk, tender
  white part only, finely sliced
1 tbsp Thai red curry paste
1 x 400ml tin of coconut milk
500g chicken breast, sliced
  into 1cm thick strips
60g desiccated coconut
1 tbsp fish sauce
juice of 2 limes
4 tbsp coriander leaves

★ Serve with a big portion of
your favourite greens such as
spinach, kale, broccoli, mange
tout or green beans.

DANG! IT'S A CHICKEN RENDANG

This recipe is traditionally made with beef and takes hours,
but I'm the Lean in 15 guy so I've used a few shortcuts to
speed things up. If you're a curry lover, then give this a crack.
You won't be disappointed – it tastes unreal.

METHOD

Melt the coconut oil in a wok or large frying pan over a
medium to high heat. Add the spring onions and lemongrass.
Stir-fry for 30 seconds before adding in the curry paste.
Fry the paste, stirring constantly, for 30 seconds.

Pour in half the coconut milk and stir to mix in with the
curry paste. Once they are fully combined, pour in the rest
of the milk and stir. Bring the liquid to the boil and
simmer for 3 minutes.

Drop in the chicken strips and bring back up to the boil.
Simmer the chicken for 3–4 minutes, by which time it should
be cooked. Check by slicing into one of the larger pieces to
make sure the meat is white all the way through, with no raw
pink bits left.

When you are happy that the chicken is fully cooked, stir
through the desiccated coconut and remove the pan from
the heat. Mix in the fish sauce, lime juice and coriander
leaves, and serve up immediately.

REDUCED-CARB
MAKE AHEAD
GOOD TO FREEZE
INGREDIENTS

1 tbsp coconut oil
300g ready-made turkey
   meatballs
2 tomatoes, roughly chopped
3 spring onions, roughly
   chopped
1 clove garlic
handful of baby spinach
   leaves
2 roasted red peppers from
   a jar, drained and roughly
   chopped
20g blanched almonds
salt and pepper
2 tbsp grated cheddar
chopped parsley, to serve –
   optional

★ Serve with a big bowl of your
favourite greens such as kale,
broccoli, mange tout or green
beans.

TURKEY AMAZEBALLS

This might be the world's easiest recipe and it tastes awesome.
You'll need a food processor for this one, though. You can pick
up a really cheap one these days and it will come in handy for
making other recipes later in the book too.

METHOD

Melt the coconut oil in a large frying pan over a medium
to high heat. Drop in the turkey meatballs and fry, turning
regularly, for 2 minutes.

Chuck the rest of the ingredients, apart from the cheese and
parsley, into a food processor along with a splash of water
and a pinch of salt and pepper. Blitz until smooth(ish), and
pour in with the meatballs.

Bring the whole lot to a simmer and cook for a further
6–7 minutes until you are sure the meatballs are cooked through.
Check by cutting into one to make sure there are no raw pink
bits of meat left. Spoon up the super-speedy meatballs and top
with cheddar and parsley, if using.

TANDOORI SEA BASS WITH CUCUMBER SALAD

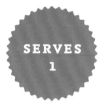

SERVES 1

REDUCED-CARB INGREDIENTS

1 tsp cumin seeds
salt and pepper
pinch of smoked paprika
pinch of ground cumin
2 x 120g sea bass fillets,
  skin on
drizzle of olive oil
¼ cucumber, chopped into
  1–2cm chunks
1 tbsp full-fat Greek yoghurt
1 tomato, roughly chopped
2 spring onions, finely sliced
small handful of baby
  spinach leaves
20g walnuts, roughly chopped

Another recipe packed with lovely spices and loads of good nutrition. The sea bass, walnuts and olive oil will provide your body with the essential fatty acids it needs and give you loads of energy.

METHOD

Preheat your grill to maximum.

Put the cumin seeds in a frying pan over a medium to high heat. Dry-fry the seeds, stirring every now and then, for 1–2 minutes. Tip the seeds onto a plate and leave to cool.

Mix ½ teaspoon of salt together with the paprika and cumin. Drizzle the fish fillets with olive oil and then sprinkle the spiced salt mix all over the fillets. Place the fish skin side up onto the grill pan or a baking tray and slide under the grill. Cook for 7 minutes without turning. Turn off the grill and leave the fish to rest until you're ready to eat.

While the fish is cooking, mix together the cucumber, yoghurt, tomato, spring onions, spinach and the toasted cumin seeds. Mix in a little salt and pepper and pile up on your plate.

Top the cucumber salad with the cooked fish and finish with a scattering of walnuts.

★ TOP TIP

Unlike most nuts, which are high in monounsaturated fatty acids, walnut oil is composed largely of polyunsaturated fatty acids. This means walnuts are a great source of those all-important omega-3 fats.

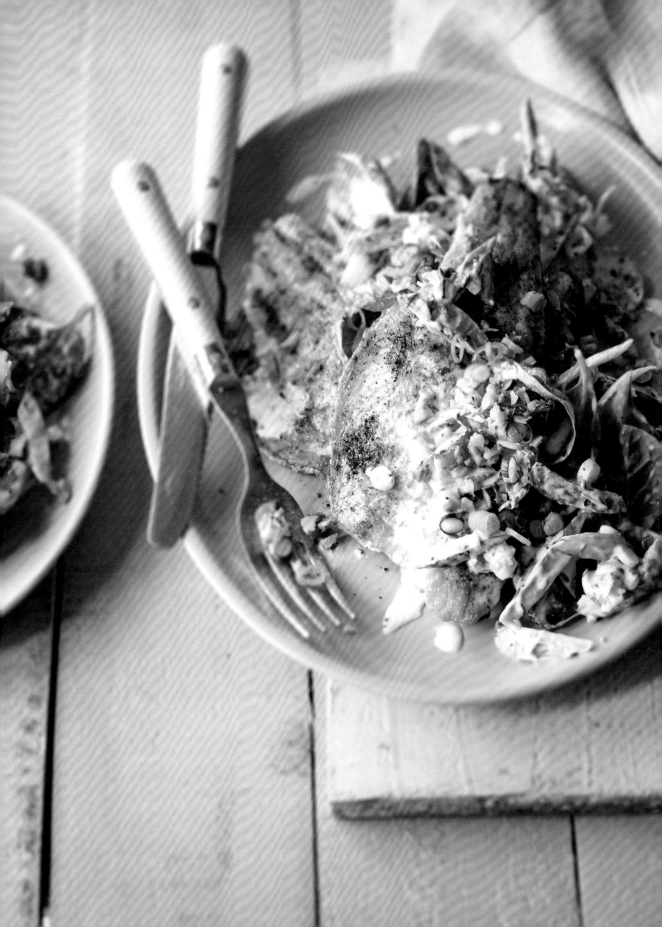

SIR LEAN STEAK WITH WALNUT CHIMICHURRI

SERVES
2

Sometimes eating a steak on its own can be a bit boring so I've made this amazing chimichurri sauce to pour all over it.

REDUCED-CARB INGREDIENTS

1 tbsp coconut oil
2 x 250g sirloin steaks,
  trimmed of visible fat
salt and pepper
bunch of parsley, leaves only
1 clove garlic, roughly chopped
½ red onion, roughly chopped
2 tsp dried oregano
½ tbsp red wine, balsamic or
  sherry vinegar
2 tbsp olive oil
40g walnuts, roughly chopped
handful of salad leaves,
  to serve

METHOD

Melt the coconut oil in a large frying pan over a high heat. Season the steaks with salt and pepper and, when the oil is hot, carefully lay the steaks in the pan and fry for about 4 minutes on each side for a medium rare steak. Remove the steaks from the pan and leave them to rest until you're ready to eat.

While the steaks are cooking, place all the remaining ingredients apart from the salad leaves in a small food processor and blitz until you have a smooth sauce. Use a splash of water to loosen the mix if it isn't blitzing properly.

Serve up the steak topped with the sauce and accompanied by a few salad leaves.

Perfection.

SPICED SALMON WITH PANEER

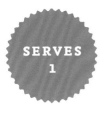

SERVES 1

REDUCED-CARB
INGREDIENTS

150g cauliflower florets

1 x 250g salmon fillet, skin on

1 tbsp olive oil

salt

2 spring onions, finely sliced

1 clove garlic, finely chopped

3 cherry tomatoes, halved

100g paneer, roughly cut into
  1cm cubes

1 tsp garam masala

large handful of baby spinach
  leaves

2 tsp sesame seeds, to serve

It's my favourite old store cupboard essential again – garam masala – that brings so much flavour to this dish. Paneer is a cheese available in most supermarkets and is like a slightly less salty, slightly less squeaky halloumi. If you like things hot then just sprinkle in some chilli powder or add a sliced green chilli.

METHOD

Bring a saucepan of water to the boil and preheat your grill to maximum.

When the water is boiling, drop in the cauliflower florets and simmer for 4 minutes, or until just starting to soften. Drain the blanched florets in a sieve or colander and leave to sit until ready to use.

Drizzle the skin of the salmon with half of the olive oil and sprinkle with salt. Place the fish skin side down onto the grill pan or a baking tray and slide under the grill. Cook for 6 minutes before carefully flipping over and cooking for a further 2–3 minutes on the flesh side, or until you are satisfied the fish is cooked through – you can check this by cutting into it to make sure the flesh has turned matt pink in colour. Leave the fish to rest until you are ready to eat.

Heat up the remaining olive oil in a frying pan over a medium to high heat. Chuck in the spring onions and garlic. Stir-fry for 45 seconds before adding the cherry tomatoes and paneer cubes. Continue to stir for 1 minute or until the tomatoes are just starting to collapse and the paneer is colouring a little.

Sprinkle in the garam masala and stir-fry for 1 more minute before dumping the spinach in and wilting it.

Serve up the salmon and paneer stir-fry finished with a scattering of crunchy sesame seeds.

**SERVES
1**

TOMATO, CHILLI AND CUMIN COD

MAKE AHEAD
GOOD TO FREEZE
INGREDIENTS

1 tbsp coconut oil

2 spring onions, finely sliced

1 tsp cumin seeds

1 x 250g cod fillet, skinned and chopped into large 3cm chunks

¼ courgette, cut into thin half-moons

6 cherry tomatoes, halved

1 tbsp tomato puree

½ tsp dried chilli flakes – throw more in if you like it hot

pinch of cayenne pepper

salt and pepper

large handful of baby spinach leaves

20g pine nuts, to serve

juice of 1 lemon, to serve

This quick and easy cod dish is brilliant to make in advance and freeze for the week ahead. Just cook it, box it up and then reheat it when you're ready to go.

METHOD

Melt the coconut oil in a large frying pan over a medium to high heat and add the spring onions and cumin seeds. Fry for about 45 seconds before adding in the chunks of cod, the courgette and the tomatoes. Continue to stir, turn and fry for 2 minutes.

Squeeze in the tomato puree and sprinkle in the dried chilli flakes and cayenne pepper along with a pinch of salt and black pepper. Toss all the ingredients together and fry for 30 seconds.

Pour in 75ml of water and mix in with the other ingredients, reducing the heat to medium. Place a lid on the pan and leave the ingredients to cook for 2–3 minutes, until you are sure the cod is cooked through. This can be tested by pulling out one of the thickest pieces and cutting it in half to make sure it has turned from raw pale flesh to cooked bright white.

When you are happy the cod is cooked, remove the lid, stir the spinach through and leave it to wilt.

Serve up the spiced cod topped with pine nuts and a squeeze of lemon juice.

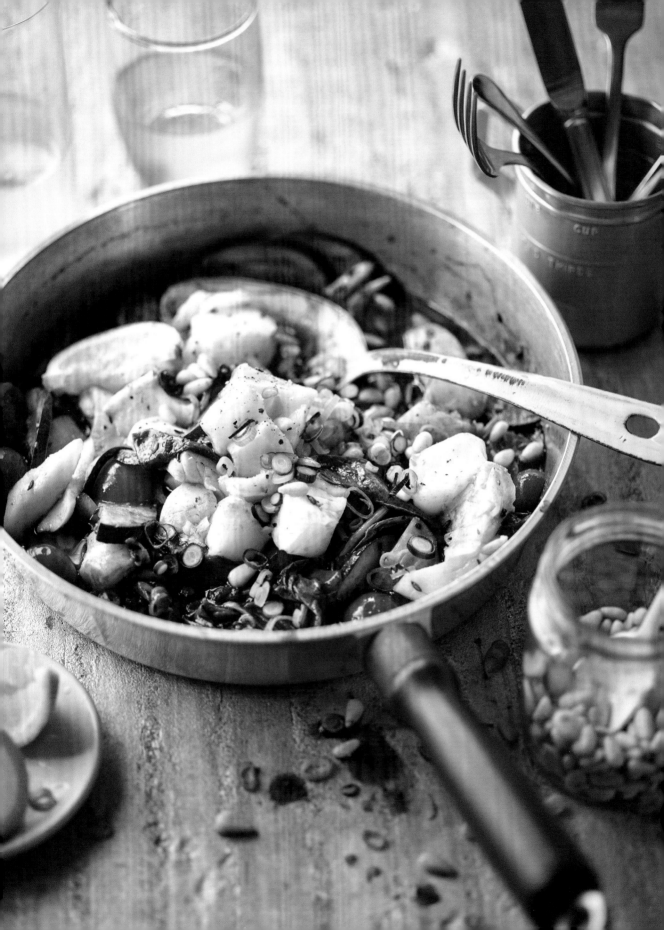

SALMON WITH CHUNKY SPICY CUCUMBER GUACAMOLE

SERVES 1

REDUCED-CARB INGREDIENTS

1 x 250g salmon fillet, skin on
drizzle of olive oil
salt and pepper
½ avocado, de-stoned
¼ cucumber, sliced into small
  1cm pieces
1 red chilli, finely chopped –
  remove the seeds if you don't
  like it hot
2 tbsp coconut yoghurt
½ tsp nigella seeds
½ tsp cumin seeds
juice of ½ lime
15g walnuts

The wonderfully named nigella seeds are a brilliant and now easy-to-find ingredient (available in most supermarkets). They add an instant and subtle onion flavour. If you can't find coconut yoghurt then normal full-fat Greek yoghurt works fine too.

METHOD

Preheat your grill to maximum.

Drizzle the skin side of the salmon fillet with olive oil and season with salt and pepper. Place the fish onto the grill pan or a baking tray and slide under the grill. Cook for 7 minutes on the skin side and then carefully flip over and grill for a further 3 minutes. Leave the salmon to rest until you're ready to eat.

Meanwhile, use a spoon to scoop the avocado flesh from the skin and place in a bowl. Season with a little salt and pepper and add the cucumber, half the chilli, the yoghurt, nigella seeds, cumin seeds and lime juice. Smash the ingredients together until they are well combined but the mixture is still reasonably chunky.

Serve the guacamole topped with the salmon fillet, a scattering of walnuts and the remaining chilli.

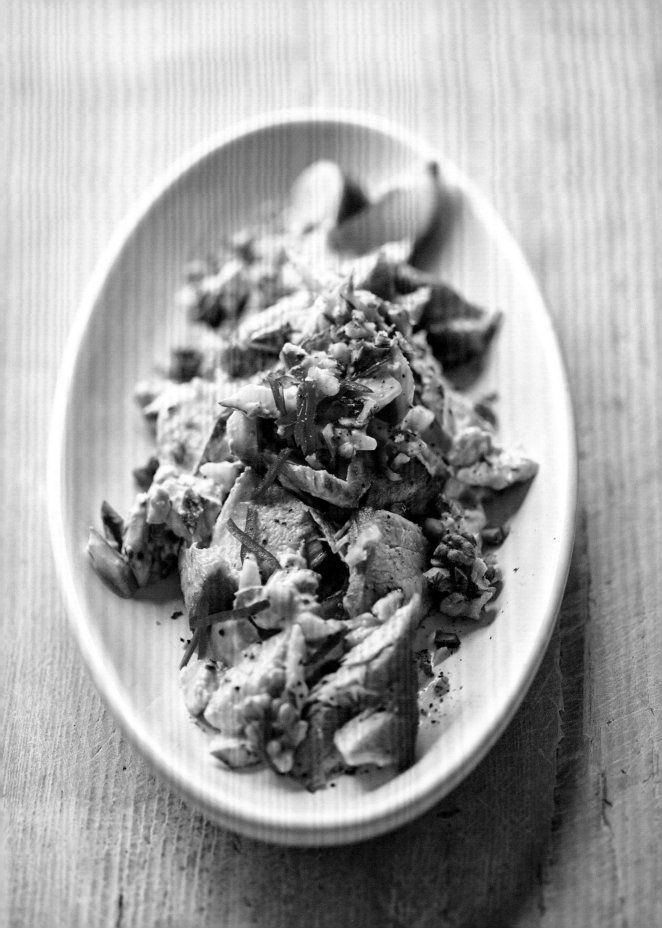

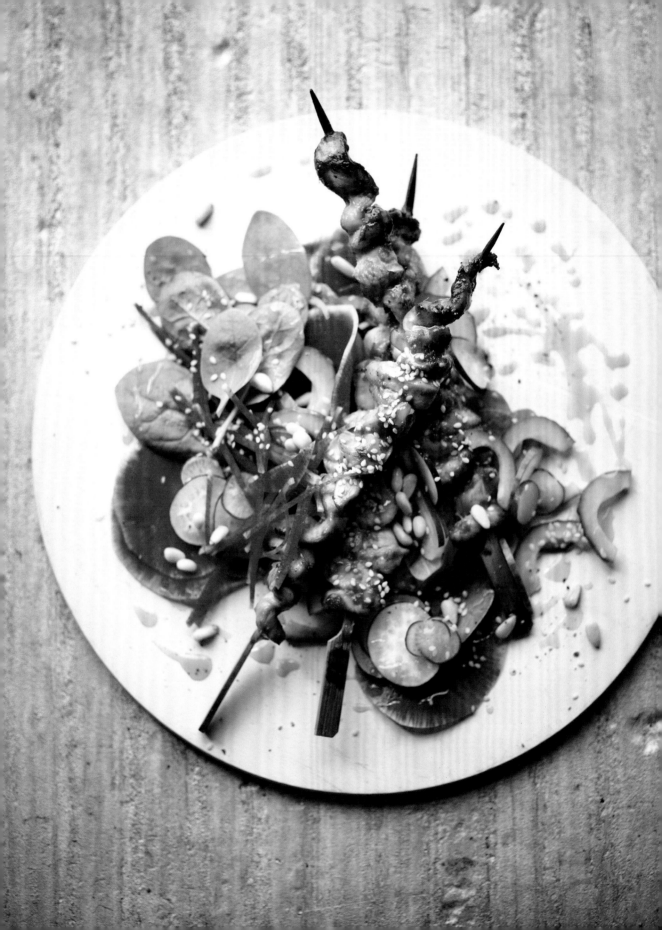

JAPANESE CHICKEN SKEWERS

REDUCED-CARB
MAKE AHEAD

INGREDIENTS

2 tbsp light soy sauce
1 clove garlic, finely chopped
2cm ginger, finely chopped
2 tsp honey
1 x 250g skinless chicken
  breast fillet, sliced into long
  1cm thick strips
¼ cucumber, sliced into thin
  half-moons
5 radishes, sliced
15g pine nuts
small handful of baby spinach
  leaves
salt and pepper
1 tbsp rice wine vinegar (white
  wine vinegar works too)
2 tsp toasted sesame oil
white sesame seeds, to serve

★ Serve with a side dish of
your favourite vegetables.

Another awesome recipe that will impress your friends as a
starter, and makes a great lunch or dinner for yourself. You could
easily box this one up for work and eat either cold or reheated
in the microwave. It's easy enough to swap in salmon, monkfish,
turkey or beef if you fancy a change.

METHOD

Preheat your grill to maximum.

Pour the soy sauce into a bowl and add the garlic, ginger
and honey. Use a spoon to mix the ingredients together.
Drop in the chicken and use your hands to massage the sauce
into the meat. Leave it to marinate for a few moments – just
enough time for 5 burpees.

Thread the flavoured chicken onto soaked wooden skewers
(see page 39), trying not to compress the meat too much so
that it cooks evenly. Place the skewers onto the grill pan or a
baking tray and slide under the grill. Cook for about 7 minutes,
turning halfway through. Check the chicken is cooked by
slicing into one of the larger pieces to make sure the meat is
white all the way through, with no raw pink bits left. Turn the
grill off and leave the skewers to rest.

While the chicken is cooking, chuck the cucumber,
radishes, pine nuts and spinach into a bowl along with
a pinch of salt and pepper. Pour over the rice wine vinegar
and sesame oil and toss all the ingredients together.

Pile up the salad on a plate and lay the chicken skewers over
the top. Finish with an artistic scattering of sesame seeds.

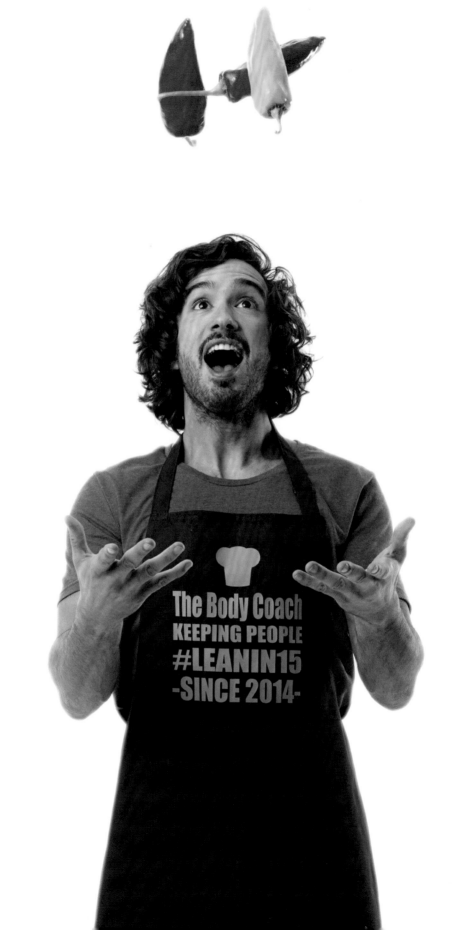

PORK CHOP AND ROMESCO SAUCE

SERVES 1

REDUCED-CARB
MAKE AHEAD
(the romesco sauce)

INGREDIENTS

1 x 200g pork chop – fat
  removed if preferred
1 tbsp olive oil
salt and pepper
60g blanched almonds
4 spring onions, roughly
  chopped
2 roasted red peppers from
  a jar, drained and roughly
  chopped
1 tsp smoked paprika
1 tbsp red wine, balsamic or
  sherry vinegar
handful of baby spinach
  leaves

Pork chops often come with a large chunk of fat on them.
If you don't like this part, just slice it off before grilling your
chop. Romesco is a really tasty sauce that goes with everything
from beef to salad. The recipe is for one person, but it makes
enough sauce for a second meal.

METHOD

Preheat your grill to maximum.

Drizzle the pork chop with the olive oil and season with salt
and pepper. Place the chop onto the grill pan or a baking tray and
slide under the grill. Cook for 6 minutes on one side, then flip to
cook for a further 4 minutes on the other side. Check it is cooked
through by cutting into one of the thicker parts to make sure
there is no pink left. Leave the chop to rest until you are
ready to eat.

Place the rest of the ingredients apart from the spinach into
a small food processor, along with a drizzle of warm tap
water and some salt and pepper. Blitz the ingredients until
almost smooth.

Serve up the pork chop with a little spinach side salad and
pour the chunky sauce all over.

★ TOP TIP

Romesco sauce is a nut and red pepper-based sauce
originating from Catalonia, in north-eastern Spain. It tastes
great with chicken, fish, lamb or pork so don't throw away
the leftover sauce. Store it in the fridge – it will keep for
3 days – and use it on your next post-workout pasta dish!

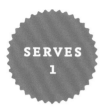

REDUCED-CARB INGREDIENTS

1 x 250g skinless chicken
  breast fillet
drizzle of olive oil
salt and pepper
handful of cherry tomatoes,
  preferably still on the vine
10g butter
3 spring onions, finely sliced
2 large handfuls of spinach
50ml single cream
pinch of grated nutmeg

POPEYE'S CHICKEN

This is one of those totally comforting meals – the sort of food that feels like a hug. Nutmeg and spinach is a classic combo too, which I'm sure you'll love as much as I do.

METHOD

Preheat your grill to maximum.

Butterfly your chicken breast by slicing into the side of the breast. Keep cutting until the breast is almost sliced in half lengthways, but stop your knife just short of fully slicing the breast in half. Open the breast up like a book, drizzle with a little olive oil and season with a generous pinch of salt and pepper. Grill the chicken breast for 5 minutes, and while it's cooking drizzle a little olive oil over the cherry tomatoes and season with salt and pepper.

After 5 minutes flip the chicken over and lay the tomatoes next to it. Grill for a further 5 minutes, by which time the chicken should be cooked and the tomatoes soft, but still holding their shape. Check that the chicken is cooked through by slicing into it to make sure that the meat is white all the way through, with no raw pink bits left. Leave the chicken and tomatoes to rest until you're ready to eat.

While the chicken is cooking, throw the butter in a frying pan over a medium heat and bring a kettle to the boil. When the butter is bubbling, chuck in the spring onions and stir-fry for 1 minute.

Tip the spinach into a colander and pour over the freshly boiled water from the kettle. When the spinach has wilted, push the leaves with a wooden spoon to remove some of the excess moisture. Tip the spinach into the pan with the spring onions and stir to mix. Pour in the cream and bring to the boil. Season well with salt and pepper and finish with a pinch of grated nutmeg.

Slice the chicken breast and serve with the yummy spinach topped with the grilled tomatoes for a dinner worthy of any table.

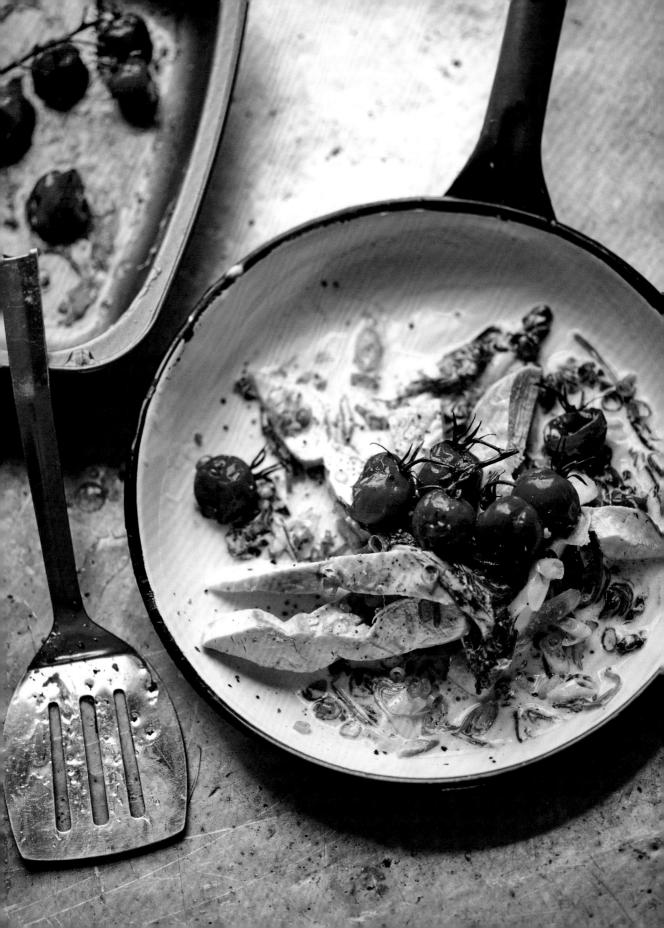

GRILLED SEA BASS WITH MINTED PEAS

SERVES 1

INGREDIENTS

2 x 120g sea bass fillets,
 skin on
drizzle of olive oil
salt and pepper
4 midget trees (tender-stem
 broccoli), any bigger stalks
 sliced in half lengthways
60g frozen broad beans
40g frozen peas
10g butter
2 spring onions, finely sliced
¼ courgette, trimmed and
 sliced into ½cm half-moons
1 tbsp chopped mint
15g walnuts, roughly chopped
juice of 1 lemon, to serve

This dish is another fantastically easy Lean in 15 but it looks really impressive when you present it. Grilling the fish makes the skin nice and crispy and it tastes amazing with these minted peas.

METHOD

Preheat your grill to maximum and bring a saucepan of water to the boil.

Lay the fillets on the grill pan or a baking tray, skin side up, drizzle with a little olive oil and season with salt and pepper. Grill the fish for 7 minutes without turning. By this time the fish should be cooked through and the skin satisfyingly crisp. Leave the fish to keep warm until you're ready to eat.

When the water is boiling, chuck in the midget trees, broad beans and frozen peas. Bring the water back up to the boil and simmer for about 2 minutes, by which time the veg should all be cooked, but still retain a little texture. Drain the veg.

While the veg are cooking, melt the butter in a frying pan over a high heat and throw in the spring onions and courgette. Stir-fry the ingredients for 2 minutes until they are just softening. Tip the midget tree mix in with the courgettes and toss the whole lot together. Remove from the heat, season with salt and pepper and stir through the chopped mint.

Serve up the fish atop the veg and with a flourish of chopped walnuts. Squeeze a nice bit of lemon juice on top just before serving.

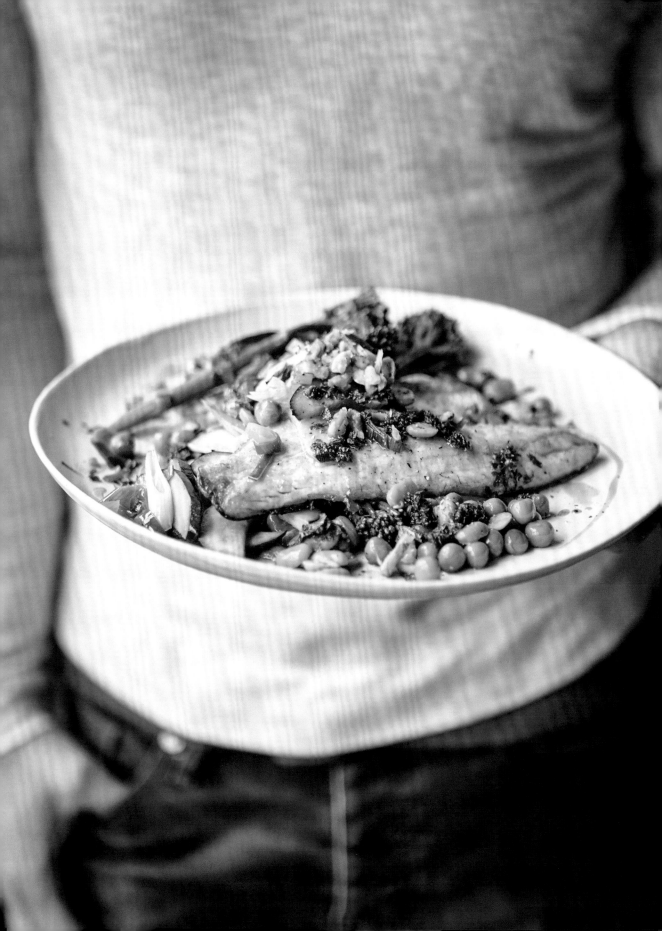

CHIPOTLE LAMB AND TOMATOES WITH SPINACH

SERVES 2

REDUCED-CARB
MAKE AHEAD

INGREDIENTS

1½ tbsp chipotle paste
1 tbsp olive oil
6 lamb chops
1 tbsp coconut oil
½ red onion, finely diced
1 tsp cumin seeds
12 cherry tomatoes
3 tbsp pre-cooked puy lentils
2 large handfuls of baby
   spinach leaves
salt and pepper
2 tbsp pomegranate seeds –
   optional

I've become a bit obsessed with chipotle paste. It's one of those things that keeps in the fridge and goes with almost everything. It tastes wicked on chicken, fish, pork or lamb. The pomegranate seeds here are optional but make the dish look top-notch, so it's going to impress your other half.

METHOD

Preheat your grill to maximum.

Mix together the chipotle paste and the olive oil in a large bowl. Add the lamb chops and swoosh them about until you are satisfied that they are evenly coated with the delicious mix. Place the chops onto the grill pan or a baking tray and slide under the grill. Cook the chops for 6 minutes on one side, and then 4 minutes on the other. When cooked, turn off the grill but leave the chops to keep warm until you're ready to eat.

Melt the coconut oil in a large frying pan over a medium to high heat. Drop in the onion and cumin seeds. Fry for 1 minute and then add the cherry tomatoes. Fry, stirring every now and then, for about 2 minutes, or until the tomatoes begin to soften and blister.

Add the lentils and spinach along with a generous pinch of salt and pepper. Toss the whole lot together until the lentils are warmed through and the spinach has wilted.

Divide the tomato and spinach mix between two plates, top with the spiced lamb chops and finish with an artistic scattering of pomegranate seeds, if using. Health has never tasted so good.

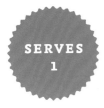
REDUCED-CARB
INGREDIENTS

6 chipolatas
½ tbsp coconut oil
½ small red onion, roughly
  diced
2 tsp tomato puree
1 tbsp sherry, balsamic or
  red wine vinegar
5 cherry tomatoes, quartered
salt and pepper
50g tinned cannellini beans,
  drained and rinsed
2 large handfuls of baby
  spinach leaves

SIZZLING SAUSAGES AND BEANS

The key to this one being ready in 15 minutes is using thin chipolatas instead of big old sausages. I think chipolatas have heaps of flavour, though, so it's a good shortcut.

METHOD

Preheat your grill to maximum.

Chuck the chipolatas onto the grill pan or a baking tray and grill them for about 7 minutes, turning regularly. Make sure the chipolatas are cooked through by cutting into one and checking there is no pink meat left. Leave the skinny sausages to keep warm until you're ready to eat.

While the chipolatas are cooking, melt the coconut oil in a large frying pan over a medium to high heat. Add the onion and stir-fry for 2 minutes.

After 2 minutes squeeze in the tomato puree and continue to stir-fry for a further 45 seconds before pouring in the vinegar, which will bubble and steam up and reduce to almost nothing.

Add the cherry tomatoes to the pan along with a splash of water. Stir the whole lot together, adding a decent sprinkle of salt and pepper. Cook for about 1 minute, or until the tomatoes are starting to collapse a little. Tumble in the cannellini beans and stir through, shortly followed by the spinach.

Cook the whole lot together until the spinach has wilted and the beans have warmed through.

Serve the sausages on top of the beany mix.

PETER PAN-FRIED SESAME TUNA WITH MINTED VEGETABLES

SERVES 1

REDUCED-CARB INGREDIENTS

½ carrot, sliced into batons
40g mange tout
4 midget trees (tender-stem broccoli), any bigger stalks sliced in half lengthways
1 tbsp white sesame seeds
1 x 240g tuna steak
½ tbsp coconut oil
1 tbsp chopped mint
1 tbsp chopped chives
salt and pepper

Tuna is one of my favourite fish, and when you coat it in sesame seeds it tastes out of this world. Be careful not to overcook tuna, though, as it can dry out really quickly.

METHOD

Bring a saucepan of water to the boil and then slide in the carrot, mange tout and midget trees. Simmer the vegetables for 90 seconds before draining in a sieve, then rinsing under cold running water. Leave in the sieve.

While the vegetables are simmering, pour the sesame seeds into a shallow bowl. Swirl the tuna in the seeds so that they stick to the flesh, turning the steak until the whole piece is evenly coated.

Melt the coconut oil in a frying pan over a medium to high heat. Gently lay the seeded tuna steak in the oil and fry for 1 minute on each side for a rare tuna steak, or 90 seconds for medium rare – I really wouldn't advise cooking it to well done.

Remove the fish from the pan and leave to rest. Toss the drained vegetables into the same pan and stir-fry for 30 seconds, adding the chopped mint, chives, salt and pepper.

Serve up the veg topped with the super-fresh and tasty tuna steak.

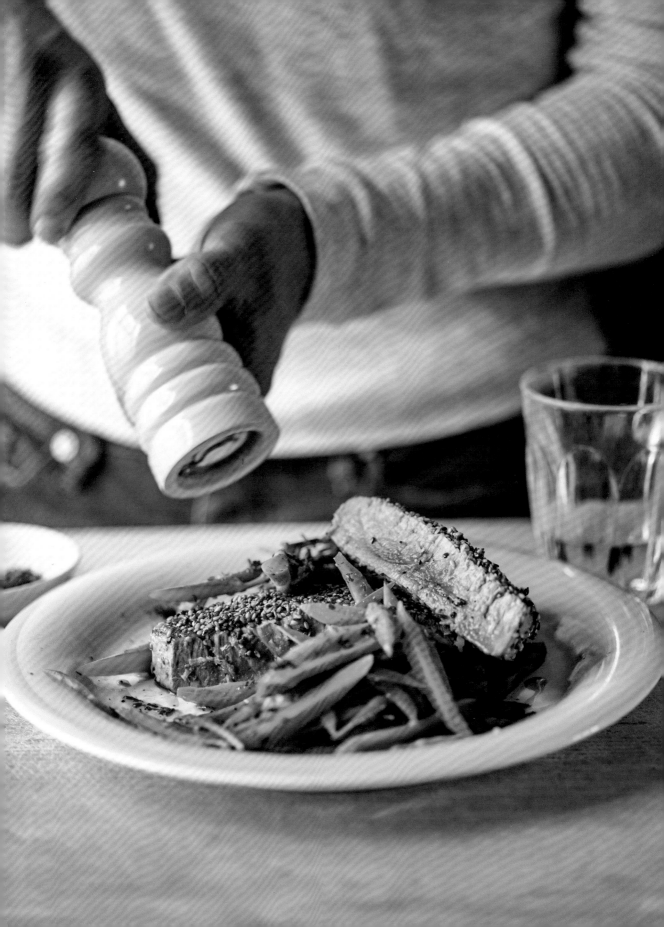

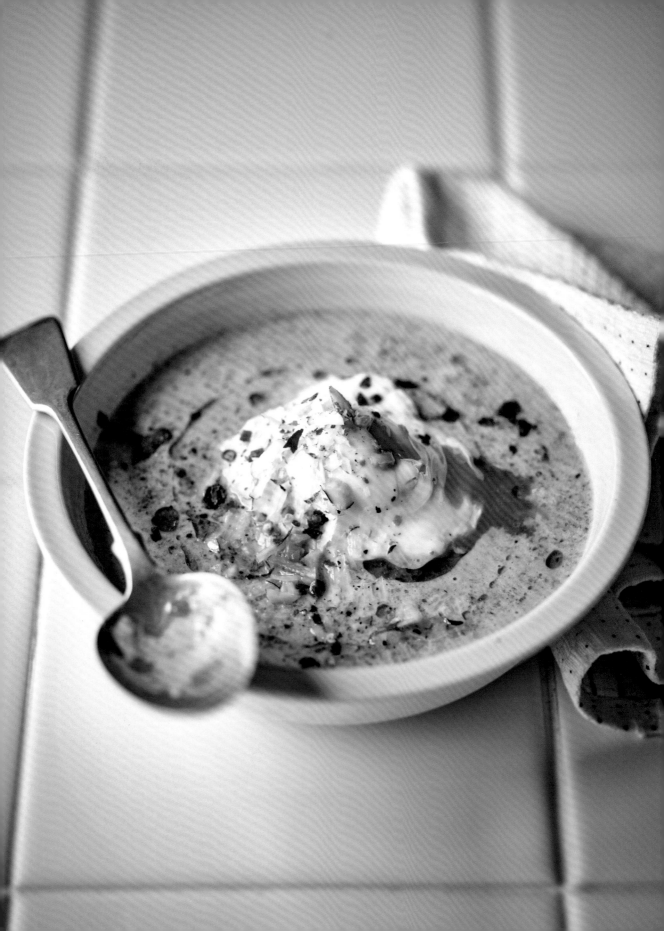

REDUCED-CARB
VEGETARIAN
INGREDIENTS

1 tbsp coconut oil
½ onion, roughly diced
100g midget trees (broccoli
    florets), chopped into
    small pieces
40g kale, stalks removed
400ml vegetable stock
1 egg
150g silken tofu, roughly
    chopped into small pieces
large handful of baby
    spinach leaves
1½ tsp sesame oil
salt and pepper
25g brazil or other nuts,
    roughly chopped, to serve
dried chilli flakes, to serve

MY MIDGET TREE SOUP

Here's one for the veggies. It uses tofu, which is a great source of protein. Even if you're not a veggie I think you'll be surprised by how tasty this one is.

METHOD

Melt the coconut oil in a large saucepan over a medium heat. Add the onion and stir-fry for 4 minutes, or until softened. Add the midget trees and the kale, and stir-fry for a minute. Pour in the stock and bring to the boil. Simmer the ingredients for about 8 minutes, or until they are very soft.

While the vegetables are simmering, bring a separate saucepan of water to the boil. Carefully crack the egg into the hot water, reducing the heat until the water is just 'burping', and poach the egg for about 4 minutes, just so that the yolk is still runny but the white is set.

When you are happy the vegetables are totally soft, add the silken tofu and spinach along with the sesame oil and a good pinch of salt and pepper, and blitz with a stick blender until smooth.

Pour the soup into a bowl and slide in the poached egg. Top with the nuts and chilli flakes.

QUICK COD, CHORIZO AND KALE

Chorizo makes everything taste good. If you've got a mate coming round just double up the recipe and, wallop, you're both sorted.

REDUCED-CARB INGREDIENTS

120g kale, hard stalks removed
½ tbsp coconut oil
½ red onion, finely chopped
¼ red pepper, de-seeded and finely sliced
50g chorizo, chopped into 1cm pieces
1 x 240g cod fillet, skinned and chopped into 2–3cm chunks
100g tinned chopped tomatoes
2 tbsp pre-cooked puy lentils
1 tbsp chopped parsley
juice of 1 lemon

★ Serve with a big portion of your favourite greens such as spinach, broccoli, mange tout or green beans.

METHOD

Bring a saucepan of water to the boil, then drop in the kale and simmer for 2 minutes. Drain in a sieve or colander and keep to one side until ready to use.

While the kale is cooking, heat up the coconut oil in a large frying pan over a medium to high heat. When melted, add the onion, red pepper and chorizo and stir-fry for 2 minutes. Add the cod and continue to fry for 1 minute.

Pour in the chopped tomatoes and bring to the boil. Add the lentils and the cooked kale and simmer all together for 3 minutes, or until you are sure the fish is cooked through. This can be tested by pulling out one of the thickest pieces and cutting it in half to make sure it has turned from raw pale flesh to cooked bright white.

Take the pan from the heat and gently stir through the chopped parsley and lemon juice to serve.

HERB-CRUSTED SALMON WITH SALAD

SERVES 1

REDUCED-CARB INGREDIENTS

200g kale, stalks removed
2 tbsp ground almonds
1 tbsp chopped parsley
1 tbsp chopped chives
1 tbsp chopped tarragon
1 egg white
1 x 240g skinless salmon fillet
½ tbsp coconut oil
½ tbsp extra virgin olive oil
1 tbsp toasted pumpkin seeds
2 tbsp pomegranate seeds
salt and pepper
½ avocado, de-stoned and peeled

I'm all about the fresh herbs and this one uses loads of them. When you combine them all together it really is healthy food that tastes incredible.

METHOD

Bring a saucepan of water to the boil, then drop in the kale and simmer for 2 minutes, or until the leaves are just tender. Drain the kale in a sieve or colander, then rinse under cold running water.

Meanwhile, mix together the ground almonds and chopped herbs in a bowl until well combined. Lightly whisk up the egg white until frothy.

Dip the salmon into the frothy egg white and then into the almond and herb mixture. Turn the fish until it is well covered – a few gaps here and there aren't the end of the world.

Melt the coconut oil in a non-stick frying pan over a medium heat. Gently lay the fish in the pan and fry for 2–3 minutes on each side, or until you are happy the fish is cooked through. Remove to a piece of greaseproof paper and leave to rest for 1 minute.

While the fish is resting, give the kale a good squeeze to remove any excess liquid and then tip into a large salad bowl. Drizzle in the olive oil and add the pumpkin and pomegranate seeds along with a good pinch of salt and pepper. Slice the avocado half into long thin strips and gently toss together with the kale salad.

Serve up the salad topped with the crusted salmon – and *mange*.

REDUCED-CARB
MAKE AHEAD
GOOD TO FREEZE

INGREDIENTS

2 tbsp garam masala

500g skinless chicken breast
  fillet, sliced into 1cm thick
  strips

1 tbsp coconut oil

1 onion, finely diced

4 cardamom pods, cracked
  open

4 cloves garlic, finely chopped

2 tsp ground cumin

1 tsp ground cinnamon

2 tsp ground ginger

1 x 400ml tin of coconut milk

60g ground almonds

salt and pepper

8 tbsp chopped coriander

JOE'S CHICKEN KORMA

Corrr chicken korma? Now that's a bit of me. This is a
proper addictive one that you'll want to eat two or three
days a week. If you're not into chicken, you could use
tofu or prawns instead.

METHOD

Sprinkle half of the garam masala over the sliced chicken
pieces, mix well and leave to one side.

Melt the coconut oil in a large frying pan over a high heat and
chuck in the onion and cardamom pods. Fry for 2 minutes,
stirring regularly. Add the garlic and continue stir-frying for
a further minute.

Sprinkle in the ground cumin, cinnamon, ginger and remaining
garam masala. Stir-fry the whole lot together for 1 minute. If
you feel the ingredients are burning, don't reduce the heat, just
pour in a few splashes of water. After 1 minute pour in the
coconut milk and bring to the boil.

Let the coconut milk simmer for 1 minute before dropping in
the chicken strips, bringing it back up to the boil and leaving
to simmer for a further 5–6 minutes, by which time the chicken
should be cooked through. Check by slicing into one of the
larger pieces to make sure the meat is white all the way
through, with no raw pink bits left.

Stir in the ground almonds, season generously with salt and
pepper and finish with the chopped coriander.

Eat straight away, or cool and keep for another time.

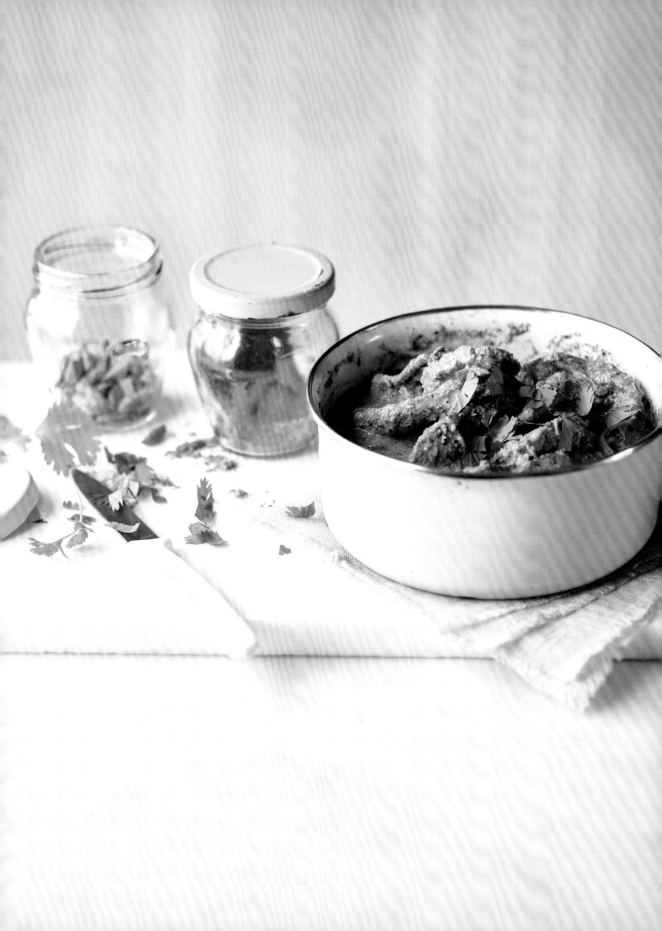

MY LEAN LUNCH BOX WITH CHICKEN

REDUCED-CARB
MAKE AHEAD

INGREDIENTS

1 orange
½ red onion, finely chopped
1 tbsp chopped coriander
1 tsp dried oregano
3 tsp chipotle paste
1 x 240g skinless chicken breast fillet
1 avocado, de-stoned and peeled
salt and pepper
1 red chilli, finely sliced – remove the seeds if you don't like it hot
juice of 1 lime
20g walnuts, roughly chopped
green salad, to serve

This is great under the grill indoors in 15 minutes but it's also a good one for the BBQ. Leave the chicken overnight in the orange and oregano to marinate and then stick it on the barbie the next day.

METHOD

Preheat your grill to maximum.

Squeeze half of the orange into one bowl and the other half into a second. Add the onion and coriander to one bowl and leave to one side. Sprinkle the dried oregano into the second bowl and mix in the chipotle paste.

Place the chicken breast between two pieces of either cling film or baking parchment and then, using a rolling pin, saucepan or any other blunt instrument, smash it until it is about 1cm thick. Unravel the battered chicken from the cling film and slosh it about in the oregano and chipotle paste mix.

Plonk the breast onto the grill pan or a baking tray and cook under the hot grill for 6 minutes on one side, then flip over and cook for a further 4 minutes, or until you are happy the chicken is fully cooked through. Check by slicing into the thickest part to make sure the meat is white all the way through, with no raw pink bits left.

Meanwhile, drain the orange juice from the bowl with the onion and coriander. Add the avocado flesh to the bowl along with a good pinch of salt and pepper, half the chilli and a squeeze of lime. Using the back of a fork, smash the avocado and mix all the ingredients together until well combined.

Slice the chicken breast and serve with the guacamole, a scattering of walnut pieces and the remaining chilli, and a green salad.

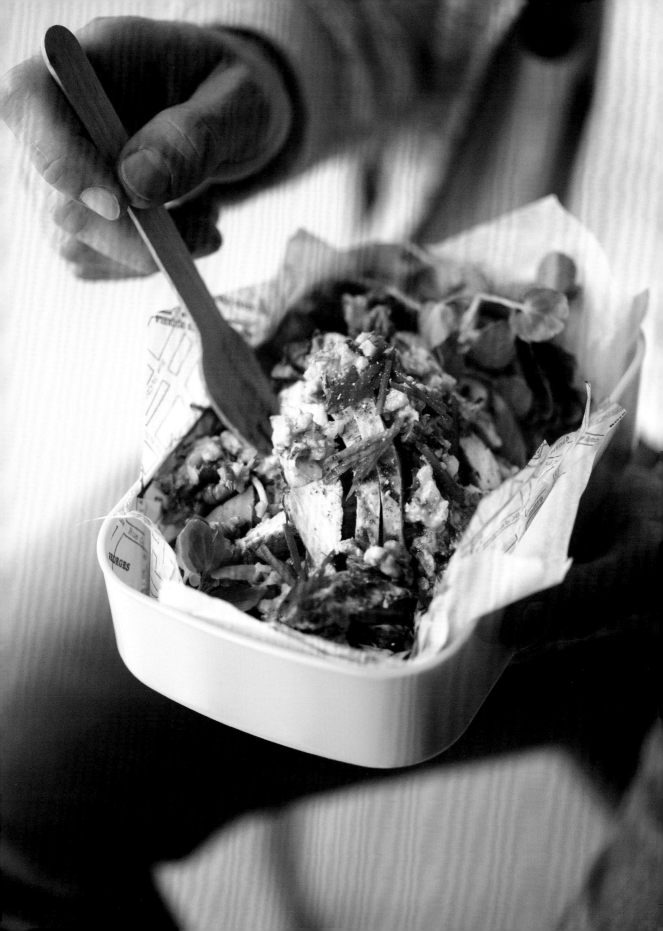

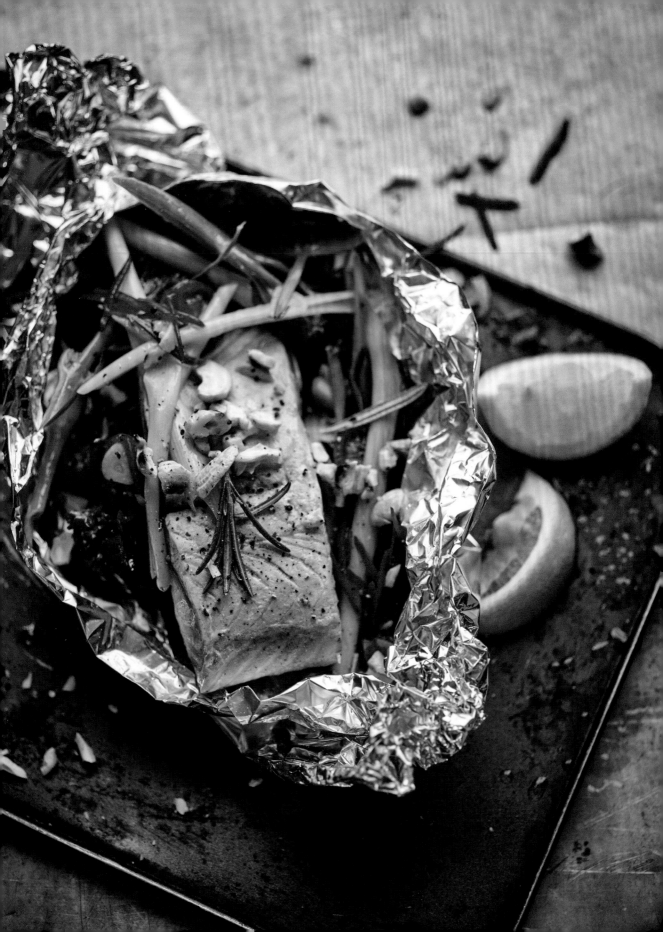

FISH IN A BAG #BOSH

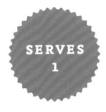

SERVES 1

This one takes a bit longer than 15 minutes but you will forgive me once you've tasted it. My PB for this meal is 17 minutes – 7 mins prep and 10 mins cooking time. I've gone Italian with my flavourings but an Asian twist is really easy if you use some light soy sauce, ginger, spring onions and sesame oil instead.

REDUCED-CARB
LONGER RECIPE

INGREDIENTS

1 sprig of rosemary, leaves only

1 red chilli, finely sliced – remove the seeds if you don't like it hot

1 clove garlic, chopped

4 cherry tomatoes, halved

3 midget trees (tender-stem broccoli), cut in half lengthways

2 spring onions, halved

1 tbsp olive oil

salt and pepper

1 x 250g skinless salmon fillet, skin removed

50ml chicken, fish or vegetable stock

20g roasted cashew nuts, roughly chopped

juice of 1 lemon

METHOD

Preheat your oven to 210°C (fan 190°C, gas mark 6½).

Place the rosemary leaves, chilli, garlic, cherry tomatoes, midget trees and spring onions in a bowl, drizzle with half the olive oil and season with salt and pepper.

Cut off a large piece of foil (approx 40 x 20cm) and lay on a baking tray. Pile up the seasoned vegetables in the middle of the foil and lay the salmon fillet on top. Pull up the sides around the fish and veg to 'cup' them. Carefully pour over the stock and continue to draw the foil up so that the edges join.

Tightly fold the foil edges over each other to seal the ingredients into the package. Slide the parcel into the oven and bake for 11 minutes. The parcel will expand with hot air and steam so let it rest for 2 minutes out of the oven before very carefully* slicing into the foil to reveal a perfectly cooked fish supper in a bag.

Scatter over the chopped cashews and finish with a squeeze of lemon juice before tucking straight in.

* Be really careful when cutting into the parcel as the first slice will release a very hot puff of steam that could burn.

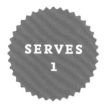

REDUCED-CARB
LONGER RECIPE
INGREDIENTS

3 portobello mushrooms
1–2 tbsp olive oil
salt and pepper
2 spring onions, finely sliced
1 clove garlic, finely chopped
1 x 240g skinless chicken
  breast fillet, sliced into 2cm
  cubes
2 large handfuls of baby
  spinach leaves
60g cheddar, grated
handful of cherry tomatoes,
  on the vine
1 tbsp pumpkin seeds

CHEESY CHICKEN MUSHROOMS

Remember I said some meals will take a bit longer than my famous 15 minutes? This is one of them – it takes 40 minutes in total, which includes all of the prep work.

METHOD

Preheat your oven to 190°C (fan 170°C, gas mark 5).

Take each mushroom, snap off the stalk and discard. Lay the mushrooms skin side down on a baking tray, drizzle with a little of the olive oil and add a generous pinch of salt and pepper. Slide the mushrooms into the oven and bake for 10 minutes.

While the mushrooms are cooking, heat up another drizzle of the olive oil in a large frying pan over a medium to high heat. Drop in the spring onions, garlic and chicken and stir-fry for 3–4 minutes, by which time the chicken should be cooked. Check by slicing into one of the larger pieces to make sure the meat is white all the way through, with no raw pink bits left.

Bundle in the spinach and toss together with the rest of the ingredients until wilted. Remove from the heat and sprinkle on the cheddar and a pinch of salt and pepper. Stir the mixture until the cheese is well combined with the other ingredients.

Take the mushrooms from the oven and pile the chicken and spinach mix on top – it doesn't matter if some of the mix spills over the side; you can scrape this up after they've been baked. Add the cherry tomatoes and drizzle with a little more olive oil. Slide the baking tray back into the oven for a further 8–10 minutes.

Meanwhile, toast the pumpkin seeds in a dry frying pan for 1–2 minutes over a high heat. Plate up the mushrooms topped with the tomatoes and pumpkin seeds – sheer bliss.

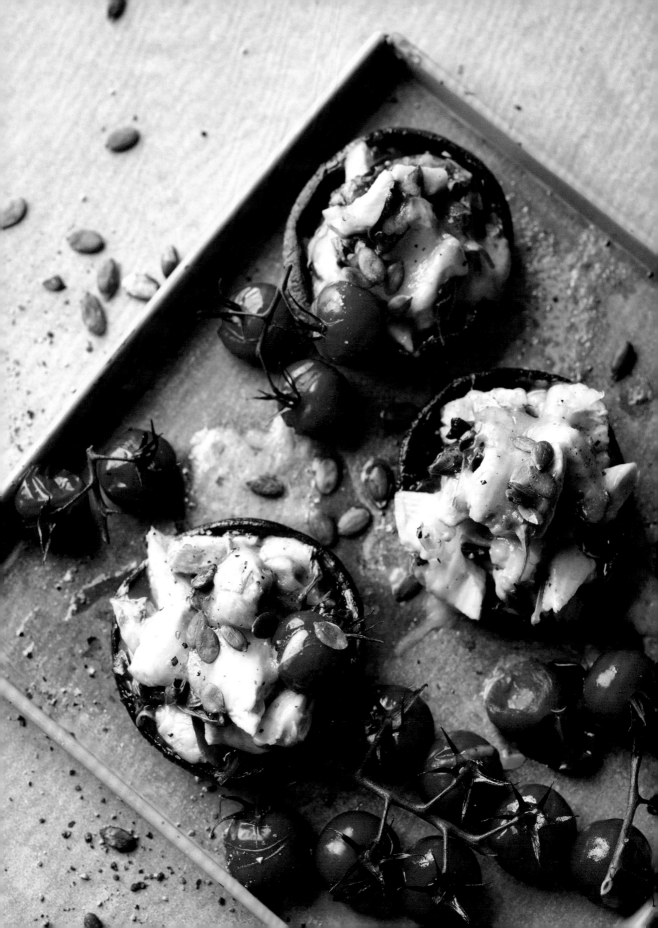

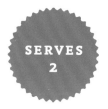

SERVES 2

REDUCED-CARB
LONGER RECIPE

INGREDIENTS

1 tbsp coconut oil
half a head of cauliflower,
  florets only (about 350g)
1 large carrot, sliced into thin
  half-moons
1 tsp garam masala
½ tsp turmeric
½ tsp ground cumin
salt and pepper
8 cherry tomatoes
2 x 250g skinless salmon fillets
½ cucumber
3 tbsp full-fat Greek yoghurt
2 tsp chopped mint plus a few
  leaves for garnish

ROAST SPICED CAULIFLOWER WITH SALMON

This is the perfect date-night dinner and will only take 40 minutes. There's a bit of prep work involved but all the cooking happens in one roasting tray so you can light some candles, turn on the Marvin Gaye and get smooching until it's ready.

METHOD

Preheat your oven to 200°C (fan 180°C, gas mark 6).

Dollop the coconut oil onto a roasting tray and place in the oven for 10 minutes.

When the oil has melted, remove the tray from the oven and drop in the cauliflower florets and carrot slices. Slide the tray back in the oven for a further 10 minutes.

While the vegetables are roasting, mix together the spices in a small bowl and add a pinch of salt and pepper.

When the cauliflower and carrots are ready, remove the tray from the oven and tumble over the cherry tomatoes. Sprinkle the spice mixture over the vegetables and gently toss to coat (I find a wooden spoon in each hand works best). Lay the salmon fillets on top of the vegetables, season with a little salt and pepper and slide the tray back into the oven.

Roast for a further 12 minutes, by which time the vegetables will be perfectly roasted and the fish cooked through.

Meanwhile, grate the cucumber and then squeeze the flesh between your hands to remove as much excess moisture as possible. Drop the cucumber into a bowl and add the yoghurt, chopped mint and a generous pinch of salt and pepper. Mix the ingredients together until fully combined.

Serve up the spicy roasted vegetables and salmon with a generous dollop of the cooling cucumber sauce and mint leaves to finish.

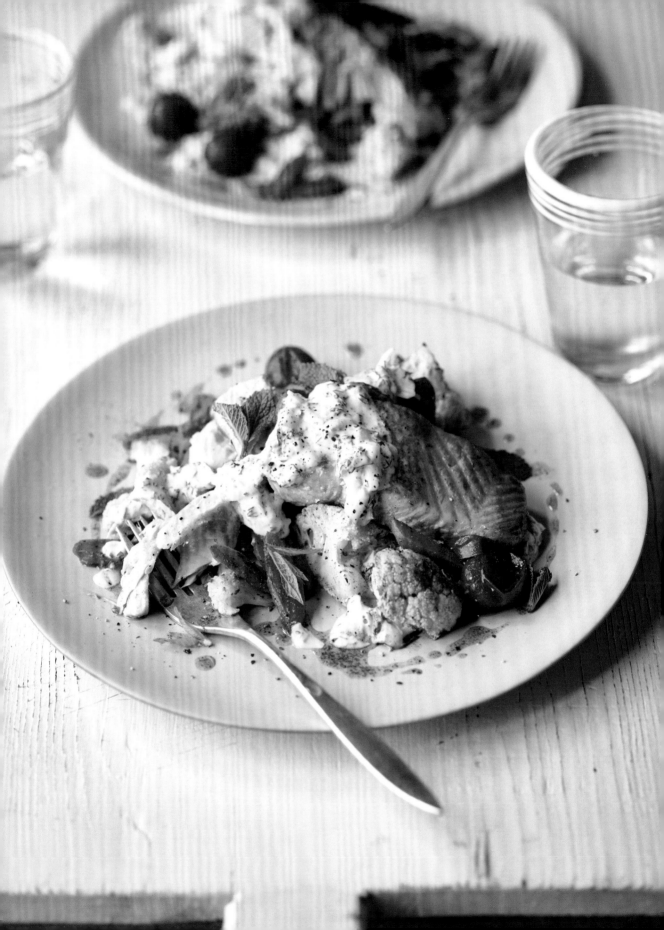

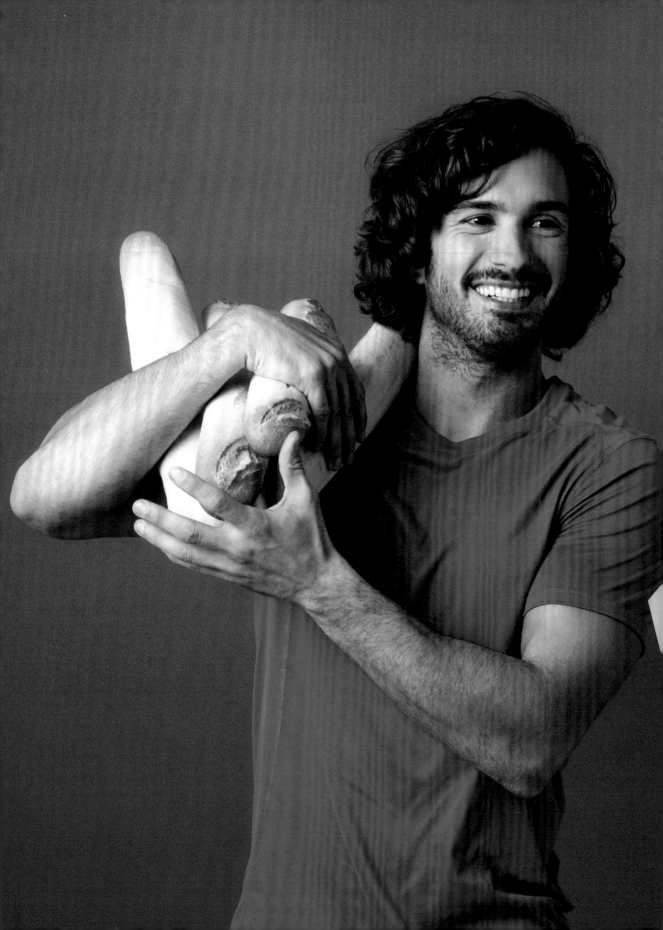

CARBOHYDRATE-RICH RECIPES

4

WINNER'S PROTEIN PANCAKES 2.0

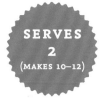

**SERVES
2
(MAKES 10–12)**

CARB-RICH
GOOD TO FREEZE
INGREDIENTS

50g ricotta
100g rolled oats
175ml almond milk
2 tbsp plain flour
½ banana
1 scoop (30g) chocolate
   protein powder
¼ tsp bicarbonate of soda
1 tbsp coconut oil
raspberries, to serve
full-fat Greek yoghurt,
   to serve
a few mint leaves, to
   decorate – optional

If you know a bit about me you'll know I love pancakes and chocolate. So here I am back with another banging pancake recipe to go with the one in the first book. Serve this up with raspberries and a dollop of Greek yoghurt for a perfect post-workout breakfast.

METHOD

Place all the ingredients apart from the coconut oil, raspberries and Greek yoghurt in a blender and blitz until you have a smooth batter.

Melt a small amount of coconut oil in a non-stick frying pan over a medium to high heat. Pour in small pools of batter (roughly 4 tablespoons each). I normally fit three in the pan at a time.

Fry the pancakes for about 90 seconds before flipping and cooking for a further 90 seconds – you will know when it is time to flip because little bubbles will appear, not only on the edges of the pancake but also in the middle.

Place the cooked pancakes onto a piece of greaseproof paper and continue cooking until all the batter is used up.

When ready to serve, stack up the pancakes and top with the raspberries and yoghurt – I like to mash mine together and save a few raspberries to scatter on top along with a few fresh mint leaves. Another Body Coach win.

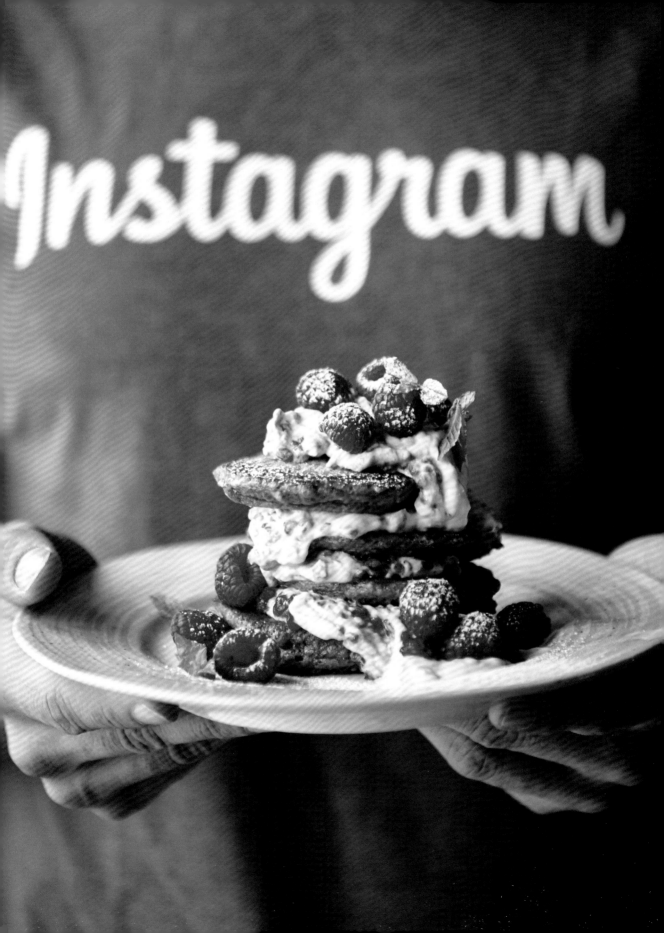

BEETROOT AND RASPBERRY SMOOTHIE

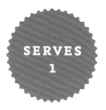

SERVES 1

CARB-RICH INGREDIENTS

75g frozen raspberries
1 cooked beetroot, roughly
  chopped
30g rolled oats
juice of 1 orange
200ml water
1 scoop (30g) protein powder

Beetroot may seem like an odd thing to throw into a smoothie but don't knock it until you've tried it. It tastes great when mixed with the frozen raspberries and it's packed full of goodness.

METHOD

Place all the ingredients in a blender and blitz until smooth.

★ TOP TIP

Beetroots are from the same family as spinach and are soooo good for you. They're an excellent source of folic acid and a very good source of fibre, manganese and potassium too.

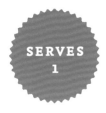

**SERVES
1**

MALTESER GEEZER SMOOTHIE

I tried to create a shake that tastes like a chocolate bar, to curb those mad choccy cravings I get. This is the result and it came out like Maltesers, which I'm over the moon about.

CARB-RICH
INGREDIENTS

200ml almond milk
50g rolled oats
2 tbsp Horlicks powder
1 scoop (30g) chocolate protein
  powder

METHOD

Place all the ingredients in a blender and blitz until frothy and smooth.

★ TOP TIP

Almonds are high in monounsaturated fats, the same type of health-promoting fats found in olive oil, which have been associated with reduced risk of heart disease.

PEAR AND CRANBERRY OVERNIGHT OATS

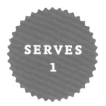

CARB-RICH
MAKE AHEAD
INGREDIENTS

75g frozen cranberries, plus a
  few extra to serve – optional
1 pear, cored and chopped
  into rough pieces – skin
  and all
175ml almond milk
1 tbsp Greek yoghurt
1 tbsp honey
1 scoop (30g) vanilla protein
  powder
100g rolled oats
flaxseeds, to serve
chopped toasted hazelnuts,
  to serve

Cranberries aren't just for Christmas; you can buy them
frozen all year round. I've chosen hazelnuts and flaxseeds for
my toppings, but go with whatever seeds you have available.

METHOD

Chuck the cranberries, pear, almond milk, Greek yoghurt,
honey and protein powder into a small blender and blitz
until smooth.

Pour the mixture over the oats and leave to soak in an airtight
container in the fridge for a minimum of 6 hours, but preferably
overnight.

Just before eating, scatter with the flaxseeds, toasted hazelnuts
and a few extra cranberries, if using, to serve.

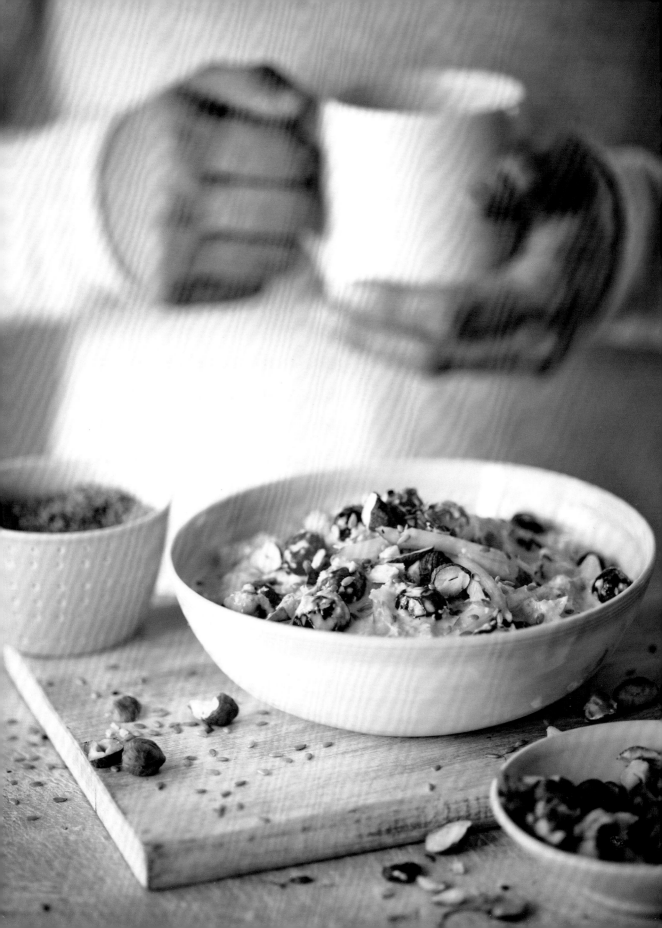

SERVES 1

CARB-RICH INGREDIENTS

1 egg
¼ tsp ground cinnamon
1 tsp vanilla extract
1 thick slice of white bread,
  crusts removed
½ tbsp coconut oil
1 banana, sliced, to serve
small handful of blueberries,
  to serve
maple syrup, to serve

OMG CINNAMON FRENCH TOAST

Yes, yes, yes. Finally a recipe for French toast that I can enjoy after a workout. I've topped mine with banana and blueberries but you can use any fruit you love. Don't go mad with the maple syrup!

METHOD

Separate the yolk and the white of the egg. Add the cinnamon and vanilla extract to the yolk and whisk together until totally combined.

Whisk the egg white in a separate bowl until it becomes light and frothy. Tip the frothy white into the yolk mixture and, with a light hand, fold in – don't become too obsessed with completely incorporating them into each other.

Dip the bread into the mixture, turning it a couple of times for even coverage. Let the bread sit in the mixture for a minute or so, to absorb as much of the tastiness as possible.

Melt the coconut oil in a non-stick frying pan over a medium to high heat and then carefully lay the soaked slice of bread in the pan. Fry the bread for about 2 minutes on each side, keeping an eye out to ensure it doesn't burn.

Your French toast should be gloriously golden and spongy to the touch when finished. When you are happy that it is cooked, place it onto a clean piece of kitchen roll to remove any excess fat.

Serve up topped with banana slices, blueberries and a final drizzle of maple syrup.

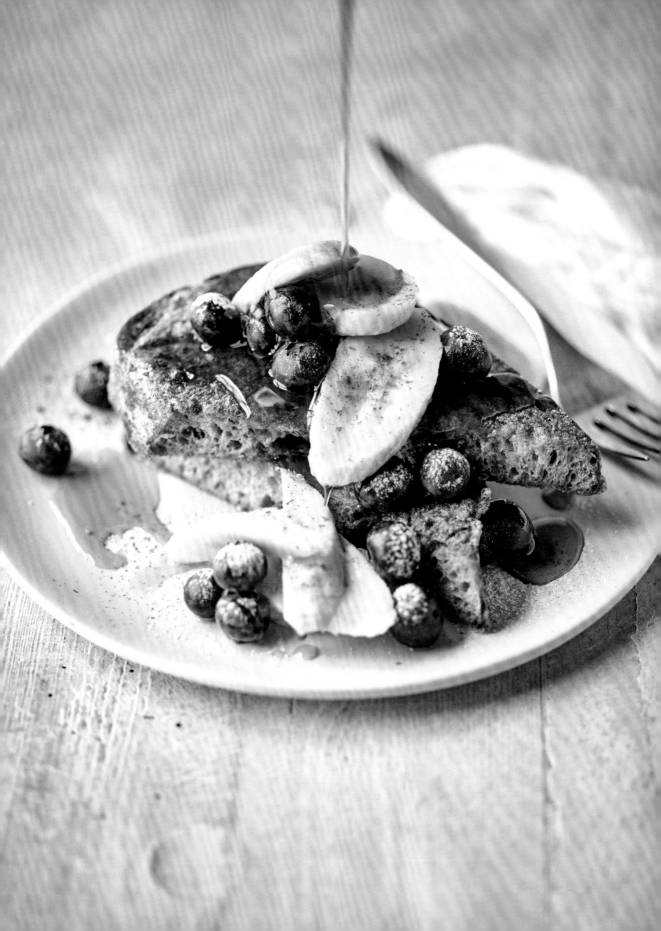

NAUGHTY STEAK BURRITO WITH PINEAPPLE SALSA

SERVES 1
(MAKES 2 WRAPS)

CARB-RICH
MAKE AHEAD

INGREDIENTS

½ tbsp coconut oil

1 x 225g sirloin steak, sliced
   into 1cm thick strips

5 spring onions, finely sliced

2 tsp jerk seasoning

100g pre-cooked rice

40g tinned kidney beans,
   drained and rinsed

2 tbsp chopped coriander

75g pineapple, chopped into
   1cm pieces

1 red chilli, finely sliced –
   remove the seeds if you don't
   like it hot

1 lime

salt and pepper

2 large tortilla wraps

shredded iceberg lettuce,
   to serve

This big boy needs no introduction. It tastes nawtee but it's got all the good stuff your muscles want after a workout. Let the lean gains commence!

METHOD

Melt the coconut oil in a wok or large frying pan over a high heat. Add the steak strips and stir-fry for 1–2 minutes until they're nice and brown, but still a little rare. Chuck in the spring onions and jerk seasoning and continue to stir-fry for 1 minute.

Next, add the rice and kidney beans, crumbling the rice between your fingers as you drop it in. Pour in about 2 tablespoons of water, which will bubble up and steam – this will help warm through the rice and beans. Stir the ingredients for about 2 minutes until the rice is fully broken up and warmed through, separating any clumps with a wooden spoon. Remove the pan from the heat and stir through 1 tablespoon of the chopped coriander. Keep to one side while you make the salsa.

Place the remaining coriander, pineapple chunks, chilli and the juice of half the lime in a bowl along with a small pinch of salt and pepper. Mix the ingredients together until well combined.

Zap the tortillas in the microwave at 900w for 20 seconds.

Construct your wraps by piling up the rice and steak, topping with the lettuce and salsa, and then finishing with a squeeze of lime juice.

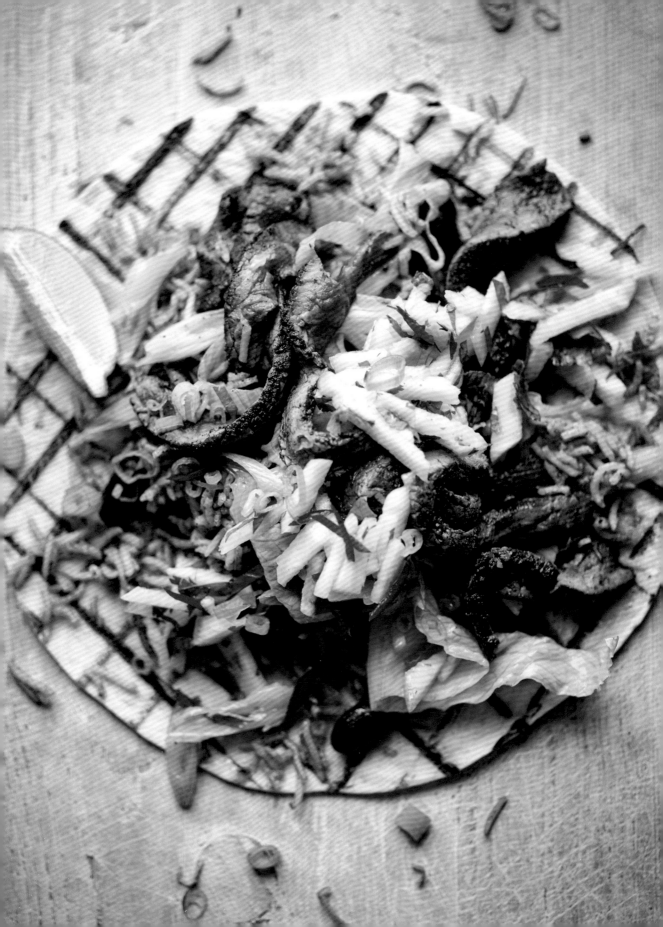

SERVES 1

CARB-RICH INGREDIENTS

¼ chicken stock cube
4 saffron strands
¼ tsp turmeric
½ tbsp coconut oil
3 spring onions, finely sliced
¼ red pepper, de-seeded and
  sliced into 1cm strips
1 x 180g skinless chicken
  breast fillet, sliced into
  1cm thick strips
5 raw prawns, peeled
60g frozen peas
250g pre-cooked rice
1 tbsp chopped parsley, to
  serve – optional
lemon wedges, to serve

EASY PEASY PAELLA

Paella in under 15 minutes? Is he having a laugh? No, I've actually done it, AND it tastes authentic too. Apparently saffron is the most expensive spice in the world. You'll definitely want to cook this again, though, so you'll use it all up.

METHOD

Put the kettle on to boil.

Crumble the stock cube into a bowl, add the saffron and turmeric and then pour over 75ml of boiling water. Mix the ingredients together and leave to infuse.

Melt the coconut oil in a large frying pan over a medium to high heat. Add the spring onions and red pepper and stir-fry for 2 minutes.

Add the chicken strips and fry, stirring occasionally, for 1 minute and then add the prawns, frozen peas and cooked rice, crumbling it between your fingers as you drop it in. Pour in the infused stock and bring to the boil while stirring, breaking up any clumps of rice with a wooden spoon.

When most of the liquid has been absorbed or evaporated, take your pan off the heat and check the chicken is fully cooked through by slicing into one of the larger pieces to make sure the meat is white all the way through, with no raw pink bits left.

Stir through the chopped parsley, if using, and serve up the speedy paella with a huge grin and wedges of lemon.

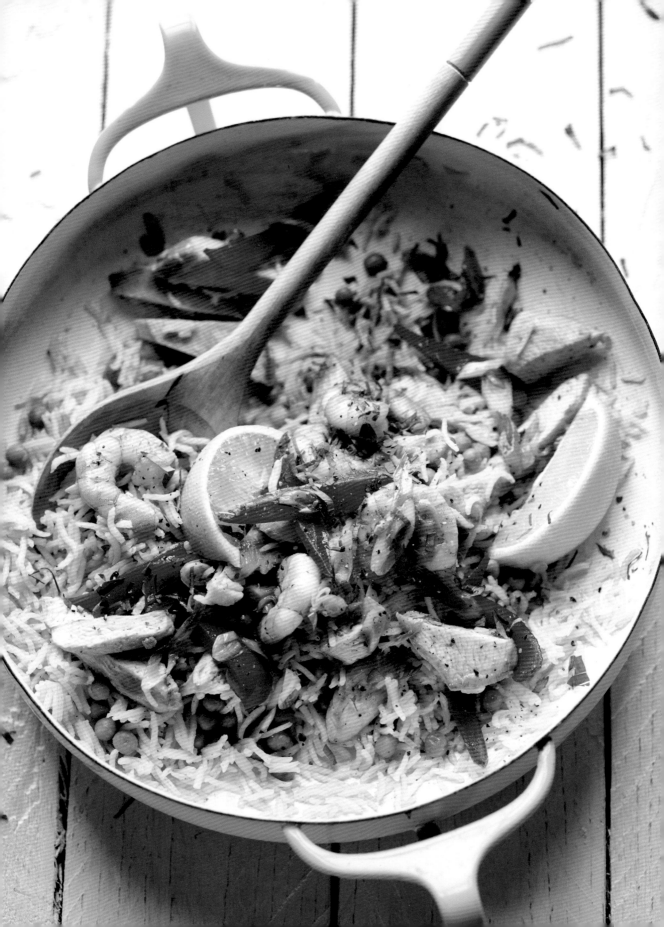

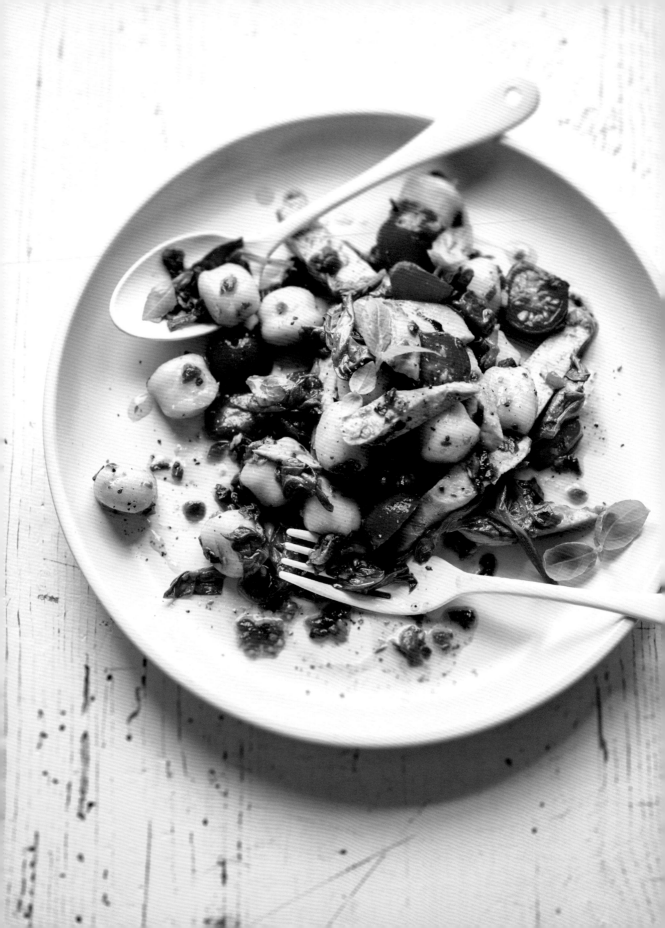

CHILLI GNOCCHI WITH CHICKEN

If you've not tried gnocchi before then give this a crack. Basically, if a potato and a pasta had a baby it would be called a gnocchi. This means it's the daddy of all carbs and is outrageously satisfying after a big workout.

CARB-RICH INGREDIENTS

½ tbsp coconut oil
½ red onion, diced
1 tsp dried chilli flakes
1 clove garlic, roughly chopped
1 x 250g skinless chicken
  breast fillet, sliced into 1cm
  thick pieces
200g fresh gnocchi
6 cherry tomatoes, halved
2 tsp red wine or balsamic
  vinegar
large handful of baby spinach
  leaves
salt and pepper
about 8 basil leaves, to serve

★ Serve with a side salad.

METHOD

Bring a large saucepan of water to the boil.

Heat the coconut oil in a wok or large frying pan over a medium to high heat. Add the onion, chilli flakes and garlic and stir-fry for 2 minutes until the onion has softened.

Add the chicken and continue stir-frying for a further 3–4 minutes until the chicken is pretty much cooked through. Check by slicing into one of the larger pieces to make sure the meat is white all the way through, with no raw pink bits left.

Drop your gnocchi into the boiling water and cook according to the packet instructions (normally about 2 minutes).

Add the cherry tomatoes to the frying pan and toss to mix. Pour in the vinegar and let it bubble away to virtually nothing. Throw in the spinach along with a generous amount of salt and pepper. Remove the pan from the heat.

By now your gnocchi should be cooked, so take it off the heat and drain in a sieve or colander. Immediately tumble the cooked gnocchi in with the chicken mixture and gently toss the ingredients until they are well mixed and the spinach has wilted.

Serve up your gnocchi topped with torn basil leaves.

SMOKED HADDOCK AND BACON CHOWDER

This is a lovely, hearty winter-warmer meal that's full of flavour. The smoked haddock and bacon are made for each other.

CARB-RICH INGREDIENTS

½ tbsp coconut oil
1 rasher of lean smoked back bacon, sliced into 1cm strips
2 spring onions, finely sliced
4 button mushrooms, quartered
200g smoked haddock, skinned and chopped into 2cm chunks
250g pre-cooked rice
60g tinned sweetcorn, drained
50ml skimmed milk
2 tbsp chopped parsley
juice of 1 lemon, to serve

METHOD

Melt the coconut oil in a large frying pan and then drop in the bacon, spring onions and mushrooms. Stir-fry for 1–2 minutes until softened. Add the smoked haddock chunks and continue to stir-fry for a further minute.

Chuck in the rice, crumbling it between your fingers as you drop it in, along with 2 tablespoons of water, which will steam up and help separate the rice. Stir everything until well combined and then add the sweetcorn and milk. Let the ingredients cook together for 2 minutes, breaking up any clumps of rice with a wooden spoon, before removing the pan from the heat and stirring through the chopped parsley.

Serve up your meal with a squeeze of lemon juice.

JERK TUNA WITH RICE AND PEAS

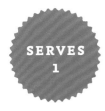

SERVES 1

CARB-RICH
INGREDIENTS

1 x 250g tuna steak, chopped
into about 6 large chunks

2 tbsp jerk seasoning

1 tbsp coconut oil

½ red onion, finely sliced

1 red chilli, finely chopped –
remove the seeds if you don't
like it hot

4 baby sweetcorn, sliced in half

40g mange tout or green
beans, cut in half

40g frozen peas

250g pre-cooked rice

2 tbsp roughly chopped
coriander

juice of 1 lime, to serve

If you love spicy food then this jerk tuna will be right up your street. And if you're feeling daring and want a real kick to it, look out for Scotch bonnet chillies in the supermarket.

METHOD

Sprinkle the tuna chunks with ½ tablespoon of the jerk seasoning, rub all over and leave to one side.

Melt the coconut oil in a wok or large frying pan over a medium to high heat. Add the onion, chilli, baby sweetcorn and mange tout. Stir-fry the vegetables for 2–3 minutes, until just starting to soften.

Sprinkle in the remaining jerk seasoning and toss to coat the vegetables. Drop in the tuna chunks and fry, stirring and turning the contents of the pan, for a further minute. Chuck in the frozen peas and the rice, crumbling it between your fingers as you drop it in and adding about 2 tablespoons of water – this will help to break up the rice and stop it burning.

Stir-fry the ingredients for about 2 minutes, breaking up any remaining clumps of rice with a wooden spoon, by which time the peas should be warmed through and the tuna cooked, but still rare. Remove the pan from the heat and stir through the chopped coriander.

Dish up the jerk rice and tuna with a big squeeze of lime.

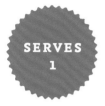

SERVES 1

CARB-RICH
MAKE AHEAD

INGREDIENTS

1 tbsp olive oil
1 clove garlic, chopped
1 tsp dried chilli flakes
1 small courgette, grated
salt and pepper
200g raw king prawns, peeled
200g fresh linguini
2 tbsp chopped parsley
juice of 1 lemon, to serve

PRAWN AND COURGETTE LINGUINI

There's so much flavour in this it should really be illegal. By grating the courgette and using fresh pasta, it's ready incredibly quickly. If you can't find fresh linguini you can use the dried stuff instead.

METHOD

Bring a large saucepan of water to the boil.

Heat the oil in a large frying pan over a medium to high heat and add the garlic and the chilli flakes. Stir for 30 seconds and then throw in the grated courgette along with a generous pinch of salt and pepper. Fry for 2 minutes, or until the courgette begins to soften and some of the liquid has evaporated.

Stir in the prawns and watch until they turn pink and are cooked through.

Drop the linguini into the boiling water. Cook the pasta according to the packet instructions (about 90 seconds) before draining in a colander and chucking into the pan with the rest of the ingredients.

Off the heat, toss the pasta with the cooked courgettes and prawns, and add the parsley along with a touch more salt and pepper if you think it needs it.

Serve up the delicious pasta with a final squeeze of lemon juice.

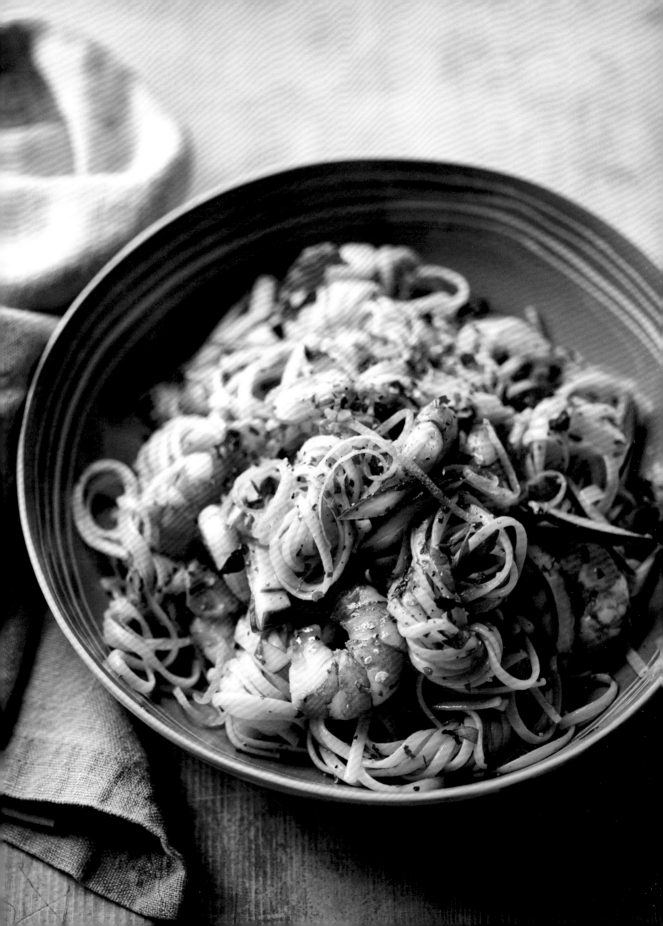

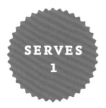

CARB-RICH
MAKE AHEAD

INGREDIENTS

1 x 250g pork fillet, sliced into
   1cm thick strips
1½ tbsp light soy sauce
½ tsp smoked paprika
½ tbsp coconut oil
3 spring onions, finely sliced
   (keep the green ends for
   garnish)
1 large red chilli, finely
   chopped – remove the seeds
   if you don't like it hot
2cm ginger, finely chopped
   or grated
2 cloves garlic, chopped
1 small carrot, sliced into
   batons
5 midget trees (tender-stem
   broccoli), any bigger stalks
   sliced in half lengthways
250g pre-cooked rice

HERO KOREAN PORK-FRIED RICE

Pork, ginger and chilli are best mates in this dish. It's one
of those meals that can be easily boxed up for work because
it tastes great hot or cold.

METHOD

Place the pork strips in a bowl and pour over ½ tablespoon
of the soy sauce and the smoked paprika.

Melt the coconut oil in a wok or large frying pan over a
medium to high heat. Add the spring onions, chilli, ginger,
garlic, carrot and midget trees. Stir-fry for 2 minutes.

Chuck in the pork along with the sauce it has been marinating
in and the remaining soy sauce. Continue to stir-fry for a further
2–3 minutes, by which time the pork should be almost cooked.

Add the rice, crumbling it between your fingers as you drop it
in, along with about 3 tablespoons of water. Continue to stir-fry
the ingredients for 1–2 minutes, breaking up any clumps of rice
with a wooden spoon, until the rice is warmed through and the
pork is totally cooked. Check by cutting into one of the larger
pieces of meat to make sure there are no pink bits left.

Serve up the fried rice with some green spring onion ends,
finely sliced.

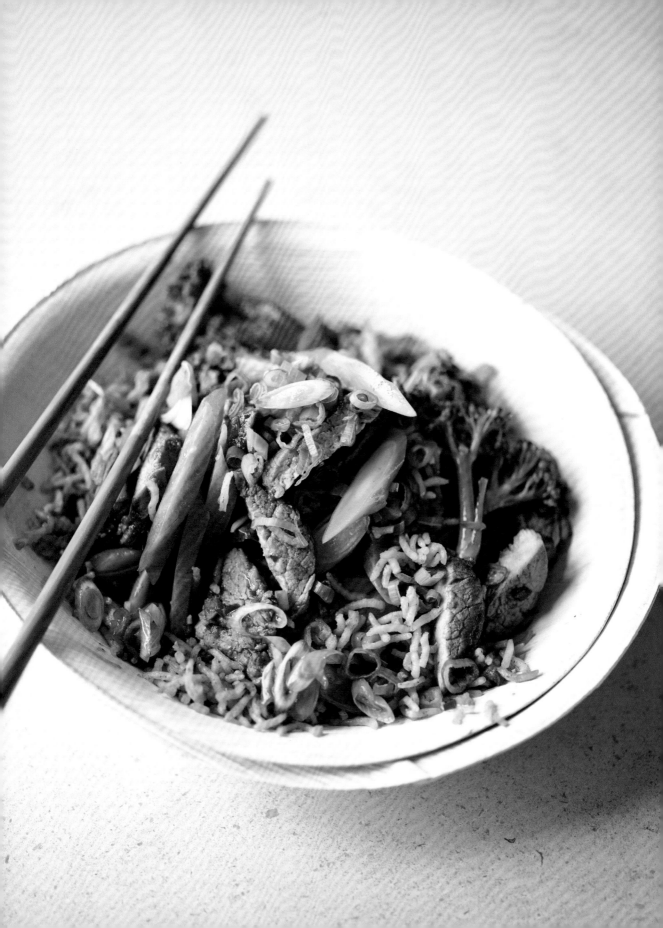

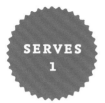

CARB-RICH
MAKE AHEAD

INGREDIENTS

½ tbsp coconut oil
250g ready-made turkey
  meatballs
200g tinned chopped
  tomatoes
2 tsp dried Italian herbs
1 large submarine roll
¼ red pepper, de-seeded
  and thinly sliced
¼ red onion, thinly sliced
1 tbsp jarred jalapeños,
  drained

MIGHTY MEATBALL SUB

I love turning unhealthy meals into lean ones like this big
juicy sub. It means we can enjoy the foods we love but
homemade and with good macronutrients. You'll need two
hands to finish off this mighty refuel.

METHOD

Melt the coconut oil in a medium frying pan over a high heat.
Drop in the meatballs and fry them for 1–2 minutes until they
are starting to brown. Pour in the chopped tomatoes and
sprinkle in the seasoning.

Place a lid (or a large plate if you don't have a lid that fits) on
the frying pan, bring the tomatoes to the boil and then simmer
for about 5 minutes, or until you are satisfied the meatballs
are totally cooked through. Check by cutting into one to make
sure there are no raw pink bits of meat left.

Zap your sub roll in the microwave for about 30 seconds
to soften it.

When the meatballs are ready, spoon them into the waiting
sub and top with the red pepper, red onion slices and jalapeños.

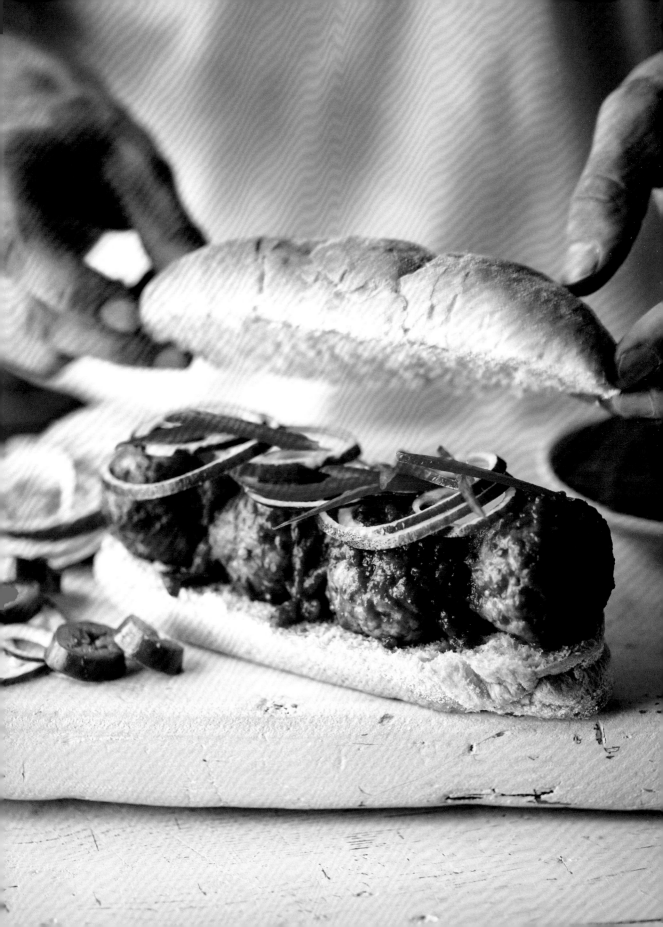

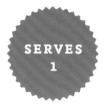

CARB-RICH
MAKE AHEAD

INGREDIENTS

300ml chicken stock

150g couscous

3 lamb chops, trimmed of
   visible fat

salt and pepper

¼ cucumber, chopped into
   1cm cubes

3 radishes, roughly quartered

2 spring onions, finely sliced

¼ red pepper, de-seeded and
   chopped into 1cm pieces

2 tbsp chopped mint

1 tbsp pomegranate seeds
   – optional

LAMB CHOPS WITH MINT COUSCOUS

Oooh I love a bit of lamb, and when it's cooked well and combined with this minty fresh couscous it's a real winner. If you're not into couscous then try the same recipe with quinoa.

METHOD

Bring the chicken stock to the boil and preheat your grill to maximum.

Tip the couscous into a bowl. When the stock has boiled, pour it straight over the couscous, break up any clumps and cover with cling film. Leave to stand for 10 minutes.

Meanwhile, season the lamb chops with salt and pepper, place onto the grill pan or a baking tray, and slide under your hot grill. Cook for 6 minutes on one side, before flipping over and cooking for a further 3 minutes on the other side. Turn off the heat and cover loosely with foil to keep the chops warm until ready to serve.

When the couscous has had its 10 minutes' soaking time, remove the cling film from the top and 'fluff' with a fork. Stir through the cucumber, radishes, spring onions, red pepper and chopped mint.

Pile the couscous up on a plate, top with the lamb chops and finish with a scattering of pomegranate seeds, if using.

TURKEY AND BACON TAGLIATELLE

SERVES 1

CARB-RICH
INGREDIENTS

½ tbsp coconut oil

3 spring onions, finely sliced

1 rasher of smoked back bacon,
  trimmed of visible fat and
  sliced into thin strips

250g turkey breast, cut into
  1cm thick strips

200g fresh tagliatelle

large handful of baby spinach
  leaves

salt and pepper

1 tbsp crème fraiche

2 tbsp chopped parsley

juice of 1 lemon

Don't be scared of a bit of pasta. It always seems to be the first thing to get kicked out of the house when people want to get lean. As long as you eat the right quantities at the right time you can enjoy the foods you love and stay lean.

METHOD

Bring a large saucepan of water to the boil.

Melt the coconut oil in a large frying pan over a medium to high heat. Add the spring onions and bacon, and stir-fry for 1 minute. Toss in the turkey strips and continue to stir-fry for a further 3–4 minutes until the turkey is lightly browned and cooked through. Check by slicing into one of the larger pieces to make sure the meat is white all the way through, with no raw pink bits left.

Drop the tagliatelle into the boiling water.

Add the spinach to the turkey along with a generous sprinkling of salt and pepper. Mix the ingredients together until the spinach has wilted. Spoon in the crème fraiche, along with about 50ml of the pasta cooking water. Reduce the heat under the frying pan and stir until the crème fraiche has melted into the water to create a cream-like sauce. Take the pan off the heat.

Drain your cooked pasta in a colander and drop into the pan with the turkey and bacon sauce. Add the chopped parsley and a good squeeze of lemon juice. Toss the whole lot together, adding salt and pepper if you think it necessary.

Pile up a steaming plate of deliciousness and gobble down.

CARB-RICH
MAKE AHEAD

INGREDIENTS

½ tbsp coconut oil

½ red onion, sliced into thin
wedges

½ red pepper, de-seeded and
finely sliced

50g mange tout

250g pork fillet, sliced into
1cm thick strips

250g pre-cooked rice

1 tsp caster sugar

2 tbsp red wine or sherry
vinegar

1 tbsp light soy sauce

2 tsp toasted sesame oil

2 tbsp chopped coriander,
to serve – optional

SWEET AND SOUR PORK WITH RICE

This is perfect for those days when you're craving a Chinese
takeaway. Instead of ordering a greasy one in, give this a go.
It's going to taste much better and it's going to keep you lean
and healthy too! #Win.

METHOD

Melt the coconut oil in a wok or large frying pan over a high
heat. Add the onion, pepper and mange tout and stir-fry for
1 minute.

Throw in the pork strips and continue to stir-fry for 2 minutes,
by which time the vegetables should be softening and the
pork virtually cooked. Check by cutting into one of the larger
pieces of meat to make sure there are no raw pink bits left.

Ping your rice in the microwave, following the packet
instructions – you're almost ready to serve.

Reduce the heat under the wok or frying pan a little and sprinkle
in the sugar. Leave it to melt in with the rest of the ingredients
for about 30 seconds. Pour in the vinegar and let it bubble up,
stirring to combine. Turn off the heat and stir in the soy sauce
and sesame oil.

Pile up the hot rice on your plate, top with the sweet and sour
pork and finish with a sprinkling of chopped coriander, if using.

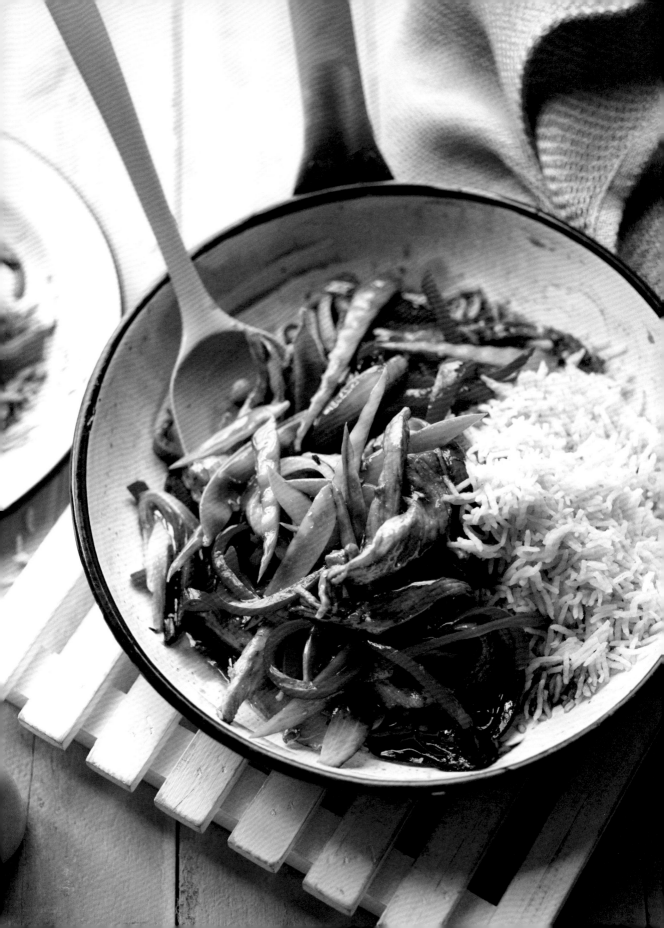

CARB-RICH
MAKE AHEAD

INGREDIENTS

2 ripe tomatoes – any type
will do as long as they are
nice and ripe
¼ red onion, diced
1 roasted red pepper from a
jar, drained and sliced into
thin strips
1 tbsp red wine, sherry or
balsamic vinegar
1 tsp capers, drained
1 tbsp olive oil
200g decent bread, torn into
large chunks
salt and pepper
250g cooked skinless chicken
breast, roughly chopped
handful of basil leaves

CHICKEN PANZANELLA

This is a really simple but delicious summer dish. Bread is
the star here so be sure to choose your favourite type. I like
to use ciabatta or sourdough.

METHOD

Chop the tomatoes roughly into 2–3cm chunks and place
in a bowl. Add all the remaining ingredients apart from the
chicken and the basil leaves.

Toss the ingredients together, adding a little salt and pepper
and making sure to coat the bread with the flavourful juiciness.

Pile a plate high with the mixture and top with the chicken
and a scattering of basil leaves.

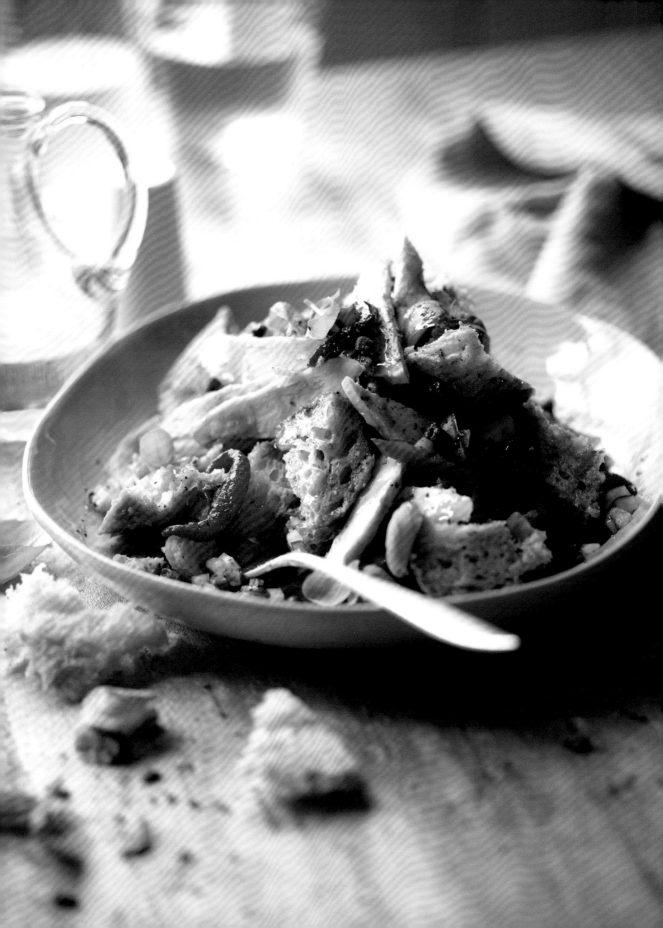

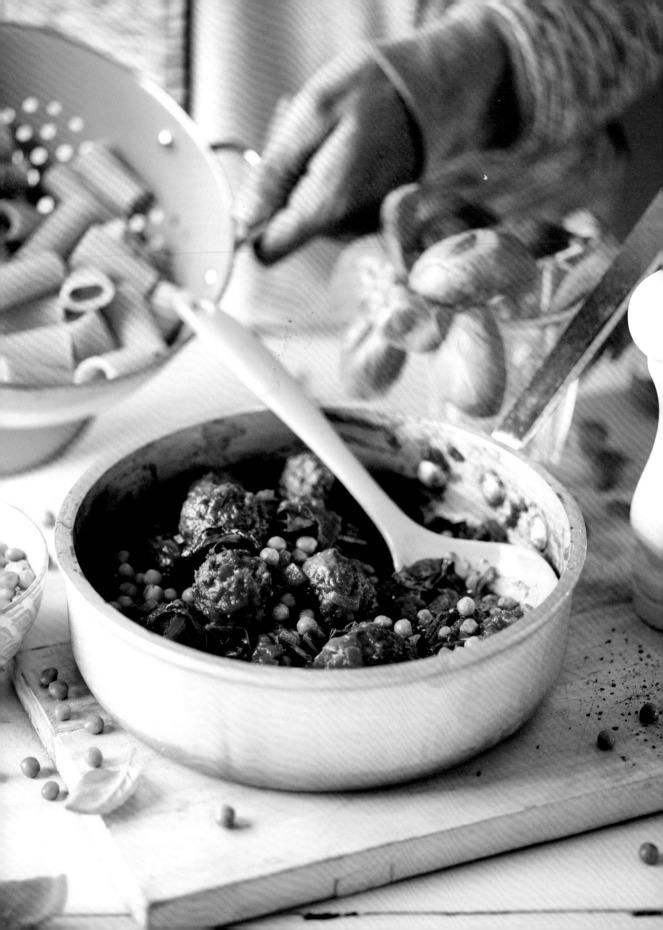

JOE'S BIG BEEFY MEATBALLS

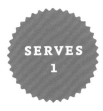

SERVES 1

CARB-RICH INGREDIENTS

200g dried rigatoni
½ tbsp coconut oil
½ red onion, finely chopped
250g ready-made beef
  meatballs
1 tbsp red wine or balsamic
  vinegar
200g tinned chopped
  tomatoes
1 tsp sugar
50g frozen peas
handful of baby spinach
  leaves
a few basil leaves, to serve –
  optional

Oh! They're back again – my big juicy meatballs. But this time with my favourite rigatoni pasta. Turkey, beef or pork meatballs will all work well with this sauce, so feel free to mix it up.

METHOD

Bring a large saucepan of water to the boil. Drop in the rigatoni and cook according to the packet instructions.

Melt the coconut oil in a large frying pan over a medium to high heat. Add the onion and fry, stirring regularly, for 1 minute before tumbling in the meatballs. Fry the ingredients together, stirring every now and then, for about 2 minutes, by which time the meatballs should be starting to colour.

Pour in the vinegar and the chopped tomatoes, along with about 75ml of water, and sprinkle in the sugar. Place a lid on top of the pan (if you don't have a lid then cover with a large plate), bring the whole lot to the boil and simmer for 5 minutes, by which time the meatballs should be cooked through.

About 2 minutes before the pasta is ready, drop the frozen peas into the saucepan. Bring the water back up to the boil and then drain in a colander. Leave in the colander until you're ready to serve.

Check that the meatballs are cooked by cutting into one to make sure there are no raw pink bits left, then stir through the spinach, allowing it to wilt in the residual heat. Chuck the drained pasta and peas into the meatball sauce, mix everything together and serve with a scattering of basil leaves, if using.

RAMEN WITH CHICKEN AND VEGETABLES

Why go to the local Chinese restaurant when you can make this for yourself at home – I've doubled up the recipe in the picture, so why not cook for a mate too? The 'straight to wok' noodles from the supermarket are perfect for this dish. If you don't have the exact veg or want to add some more then go for it. Be creative!

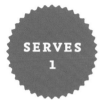

SERVES 1

CARB-RICH
INGREDIENTS

300ml chicken or vegetable stock (fresh is better for this recipe)

3 midget trees (tender-stem broccoli), sliced in half lengthways

40g mange tout

1 tbsp oyster sauce

2 tsp light soy sauce

250g 'straight to wok' medium noodles

100g silken tofu, chopped into 2cm cubes

150g cooked skinless chicken breast, roughly sliced into bite-sized pieces

40g beansprouts

1 spring onion, finely sliced

METHOD

Pour the stock into a saucepan and bring up to the boil. At the same time put a kettle on to boil.

When the stock is boiling, drop in the midget trees and mange tout and simmer for 1 minute before taking the pan off the heat and stirring in the oyster sauce and light soy sauce.

Tip the noodles from their packet into a sieve or colander over the sink. Pour the boiled water from the kettle over the noodles – this will help to separate them, warm them up and also rinse off the weird oil they are coated in. Drain the noodles well and then tip them into a bowl.

Top the noodles with the silken tofu and cooked chicken and pour over the hot stock and vegetables.

Give the noodles a few minutes to warm up before topping them with the crunchy beansprouts and sprinkling with the spring onion.

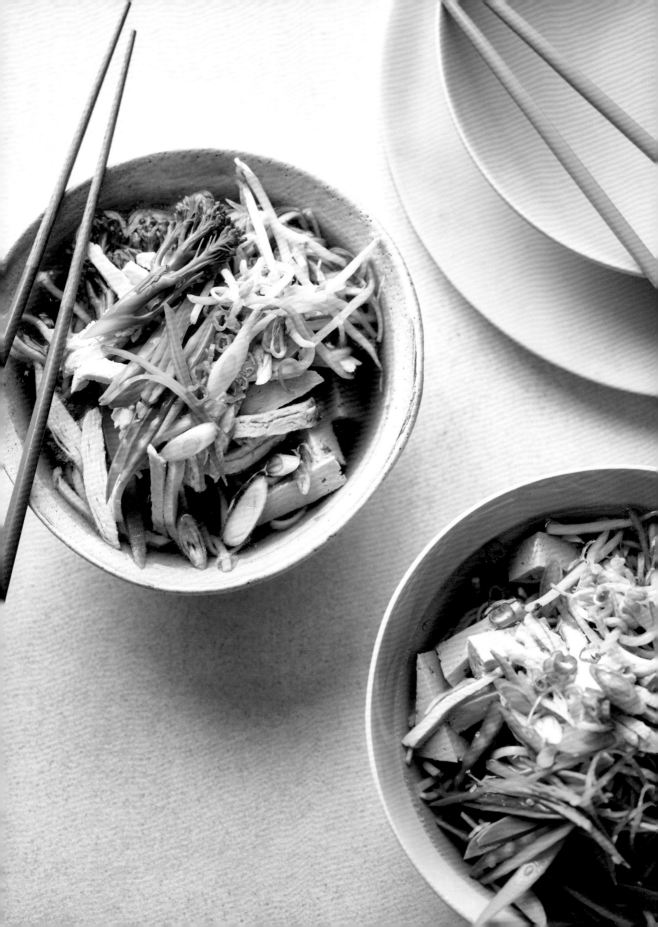

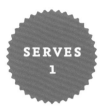

**SERVES
1**

CARB-RICH
MAKE AHEAD
(the tabbouleh, not
the kebabs)

INGREDIENTS

50g dried bulgur wheat
250g monkfish, trimmed and
  chopped into 2–3cm chunks
drizzle of olive oil
salt and pepper
3 tbsp chopped parsley
2 tbsp chopped mint
2 tbsp chopped coriander
1 ripe tomato, roughly
  chopped
2 roasted red peppers from a
  jar, roughly sliced
2 spring onions, finely sliced
2 lemons
pitta bread, to serve

MONKFISH KEBABS WITH TABBOULEH

This tabbouleh tastes fresh and healthy, and leaving it to
sit means all the flavours develop nicely. If you don't have
skewers, don't worry – just grill the monkfish chunks without
spearing them, and cook for a little less time.

METHOD

Preheat your grill to maximum and bring a saucepan of water
to the boil.

As soon as the water has boiled, dump in the bulgur wheat
and cook according to the packet instructions (about 8 minutes)
before draining through a fine sieve and rinsing under cold
running water.

Slide the monkfish onto one massive skewer or two smaller
ones (see tip on page 39). Drizzle with olive oil and season with
salt and pepper. Grill the monkfish for 8–9 minutes, rotating
a couple of times while cooking.

Tip the drained bulgur wheat into a bowl and add the chopped
herbs, the tomato (scraping in all the tomato juice too), red
pepper, spring onions, the juice of 1 lemon and a generous
pinch of salt and pepper. Mix the ingredients together.

Serve up the tabbouleh with the cooked monkfish skewers
on top, a final spritz of lemon juice, some grated lemon zest
and pitta bread on the side.

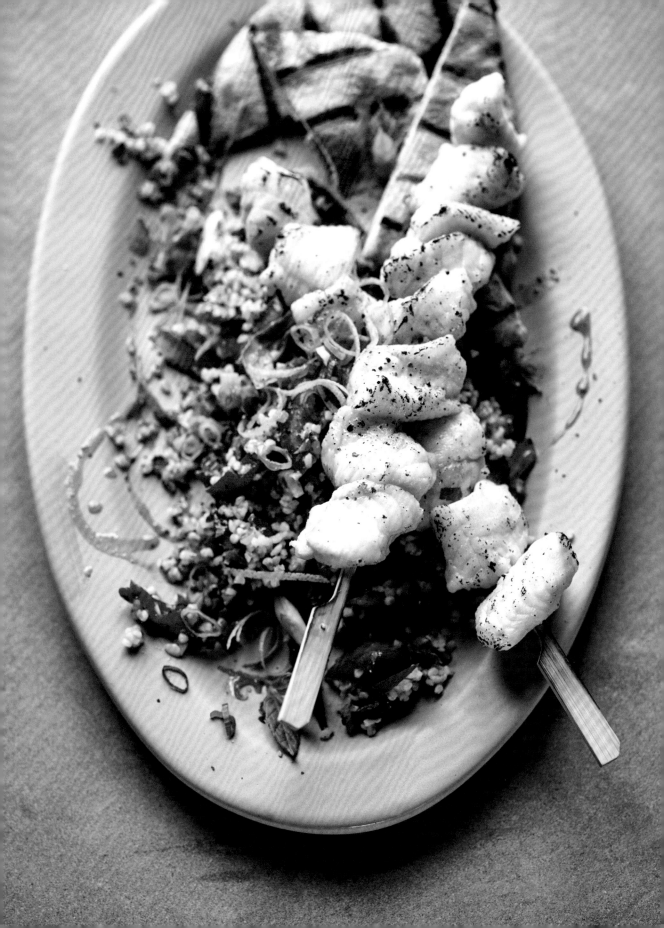

AUSSIE BUM BURGER WITH WEDGES

SERVES 2

CARB-RICH
INGREDIENTS

2 sweet potatoes
550g chicken mince
4 spring onions, finely sliced
1 egg
2 tbsp fresh breadcrumbs
3 tbsp chopped parsley
3 tbsp chopped basil
salt and pepper
1 tbsp coconut oil
2 tbsp low-fat crème fraiche
2 tsp harissa paste
2 burger buns
2 pineapple rings (fresh is best,
   but from the tin is fine)
4 large slices of cooked
   beetroot

The Aussies love a bit of beetroot and pineapple on their burgers and after creating this recipe so do I. Share your burger pics with me on Twitter or Instagram @thebodycoach and I'll regram the best lookers. If you can't find chicken mince then turkey mince works well here.

METHOD

Preheat your grill to maximum.

Slice the sweet potatoes in half lengthways, and then chop into 4 wedges per half. Place the 16 wedges on a plate, microwave at 900w for 6 minutes, then leave to stand for 1 minute.

While the sweet potatoes are cooking, chuck the chicken mince, spring onions, egg, breadcrumbs, parsley, basil and a good amount of salt and pepper into a bowl. Get stuck in with your hands and knead the ingredients for 1 minute until well combined.

Shape the mixture into two large burgers. Diameter isn't that important, but try to pat them into roughly the same thickness – about 2cm – to help them cook evenly. Place the burgers on the grill pan or a baking tray and slide under the grill. Cook the burgers for 6 minutes per side. Check they are cooked by slicing into one to make sure the meat is white all the way through, with no raw pink bits left.

While the burgers are cooking, melt the coconut oil in a large frying pan over a medium to high heat. Toss in the microwaved sweet potato wedges and fry for about 3 minutes, turning a couple of times to colour. Drain the wedges on a piece of kitchen roll, and give them a sprinkle of salt. Leave to rest until ready to serve.

Mix together the crème fraiche and harissa paste and construct your burger however you fancy. I like to spread the harissa mix on the bun, plonk the burger on top and finish with the pineapple, beetroot and then finally the lid. I advise using cutlery for this burger – it can get messy!

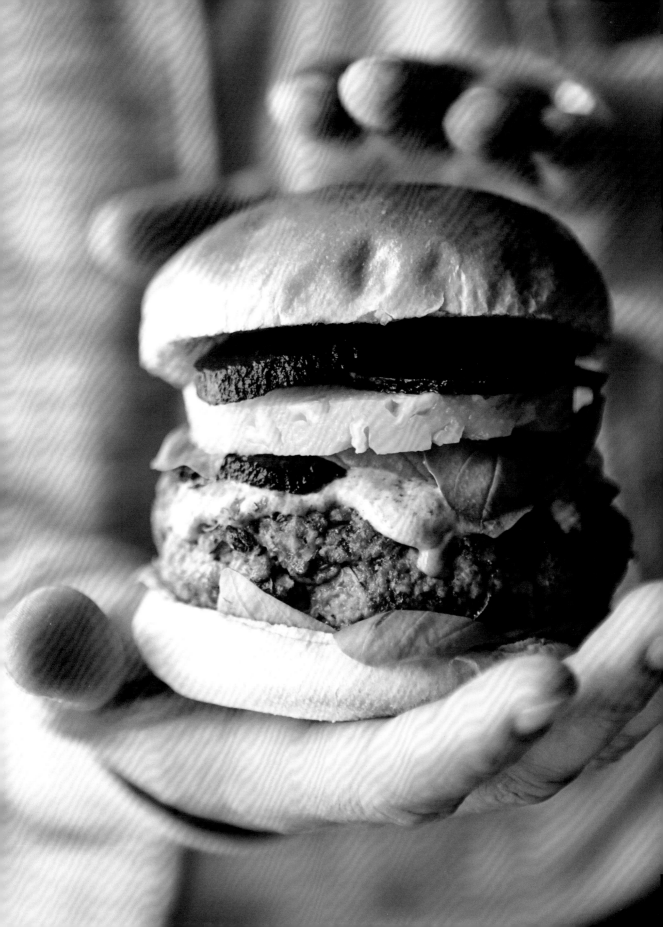

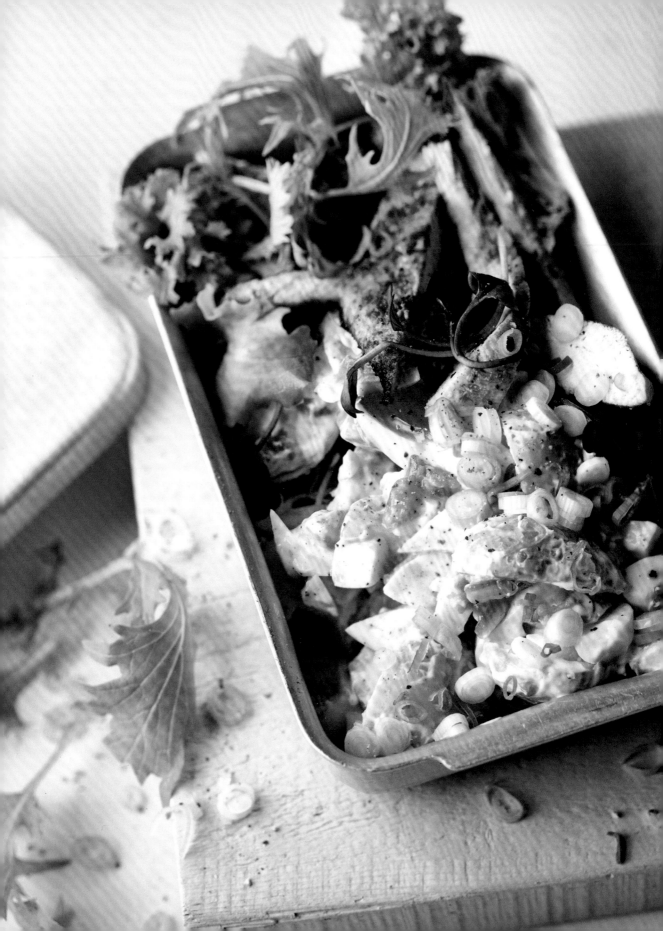

CARB-RICH
MAKE AHEAD

INGREDIENTS

180g new potatoes, halved
2 eggs
1 x 200g skinless chicken
  breast fillet
2 pinches of smoked paprika
salt and pepper
1 tbsp low-fat crème fraiche
2 spring onions, finely sliced
green salad, to serve

POTATO SALAD WITH BUTTERFLY CHICKEN

Quick, easy and full of goodness, this is the perfect go-to meal if you're in a hurry and don't fancy making too much effort. It will also go well in a lunch box for work.

METHOD

Bring a saucepan of water to the boil and preheat your grill to maximum.

When the water is boiling, drop in the potato halves and simmer for 5 minutes. When the time is up, carefully lower in the eggs and boil for a further 7 minutes. Drain the potatoes and eggs in a sieve or colander.

While the potatoes and eggs are cooking, place the chicken breast flat on a chopping board and, using a sharp knife, slice into the side of the breast and cut almost to the very end – as if you are cutting the breast in half from the side, but just stopping short. Open the breast up like a book and sprinkle with the smoked paprika and a generous pinch of salt and pepper. Place onto the grill pan or a baking tray and slide under the grill. Cook for 5 minutes on each side, by which time it should be perfectly cooked. Check by slicing into it to make sure that the meat is white all the way through, with no raw pink bits left. Turn off the heat and leave the chicken to rest until you're ready to eat.

Tip the potatoes into a bowl and add the crème fraiche. Peel the eggs and carefully separate the yolks and the whites – don't worry about being perfect here. The yolk should be cooked around the edge, but still a little runny. Drop the yolks in with the potatoes, add a generous pinch of salt and pepper and mix the ingredients well.

Crumble the egg whites in with the potatoes, add the spring onions and gently mix together.

Slice the chicken and serve on top of the potato salad with a side of greens.

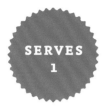

CARB-RICH
MAKE AHEAD
GOOD TO FREEZE

INGREDIENTS

200g dried orzo
50g frozen peas
½ tbsp coconut oil
2 rashers of smoked back
  bacon, cut into 1cm thick
  strips
1 clove garlic, finely chopped
2 spring onions, finely sliced
1 x 200g skinless chicken
  breast fillet, sliced into
  small 2–3cm chunks
handful of baby spinach
  leaves
juice of 1 lemon, to serve

BACON AND PEA ORZO

Orzo looks like rice but it's actually a pasta, which is a win. This recipe is good to make ahead and freeze, so you could always double up when you're prepping like a boss so that you've got one meal sorted for the week ahead.

METHOD

Bring a saucepan of water to the boil. Drop in the orzo and cook according to the packet instructions. Then, 2 minutes before the cooking time is up, drop in the frozen peas. When both pasta and peas are cooked, drain in a fine sieve.

Meanwhile, melt the coconut oil in a large frying pan over a medium to high heat. Add the bacon strips and fry for 45 seconds.

Chuck in the garlic, spring onions and chicken and stir-fry for 2–3 minutes, by which time the chicken should be almost ready. Carefully scoop out about half a mugful of the water the pasta is cooking in and pour into the pan with the chicken. It will bubble up quickly, so reduce the heat and continue simmering until the chicken is cooked through. Check by slicing into one of the larger pieces to make sure the meat is white all the way through, with no raw pink bits left.

Next, add the orzo and peas to the frying pan along with the spinach. Remove from the hob and toss the whole lot together until the spinach has wilted in the residual heat.

Dish up the pasta and finish with a squeeze of lemon juice. Sit and enjoy a warm, comforting meal.

SWEET POTATO WITH CHIPOTLE BUTTER CHICKEN

SERVES 1

CARB-RICH
MAKE AHEAD

INGREDIENTS

1 medium sweet potato
15g butter, softened
2 tsp chipotle paste
salt and pepper
½ tbsp coconut oil
2 spring onions, finely sliced
1 x 250g skinless chicken
  breast fillet, sliced into
  1cm strips
juice of 1 lime

★ Serve with a side salad.

My love affair with chipotle paste continues here. I can't get enough of the stuff. It tastes amazing, especially when you mix it with butter. Experiment with flavoured butters – they are a really good way of livening up a dull piece of meat and make a tasty filling for a jacket potato.

METHOD

Zap the sweet potato in the microwave at 900w for 5 minutes, leave to rest for 1 minute and then zap for a further 4 minutes.

While the potato is in the microwave, mix together the butter and chipotle paste along with a pinch of salt and pepper.

Melt the coconut oil in a frying pan over a medium to high heat. Chuck in the spring onions and chicken strips and stir-fry for 3–4 minutes until you are sure the chicken is cooked through. Check by slicing into one of the larger pieces to make sure the meat is white all the way through, with no raw pink bits left. Reduce the heat to low and spoon in the butter along with the lime juice. Let the butter melt and warm through.

Remove the sweet potato from the microwave, slice open on a plate and pour over the zingy chicken.

★ TOP TIP

Flavoured butters are great to have to hand: make a batch and keep in the freezer until you need it. Try combining 100g butter with 2 tablespoons of finely chopped parsley and 1 crushed garlic clove. Bosh! – you've got yourself some garlic butter.

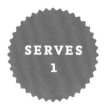

SERVES 1

PESTO PENNE WITH GRILLED TUNA

CARB-RICH
MAKE AHEAD

INGREDIENTS

200g fresh penne
6 cherry tomatoes
handful of baby spinach
  leaves
1 tbsp pesto
salt and pepper
½ tbsp coconut oil
1 x 250g tuna steak
a few basil leaves – optional

Oooh more pasta? Yes please, #CarbMe. You may already have a jar of pesto kicking around in the back of your cupboard, but if not you can always make your own at home. I use fresh pasta in this dish as it tastes better and speeds things up.

METHOD

Bring a large saucepan of water to the boil. Add the pasta and cook for 2 minutes, or according to the packet instructions. About 30 seconds before the cooking time is up, drop in the cherry tomatoes and let them boil with the pasta.

Chuck the spinach into a colander and when the pasta is cooked, tip it into the colander – the heat of the water will cook the spinach. Tip the contents back into the saucepan and mix in the pesto. Season with a little salt and pepper, cover with a lid to keep warm and leave to one side while you cook the tuna.

Melt the coconut oil in a frying pan over a high heat and fry the tuna for 1 minute on each side (this will give you a rare piece of fish; if you prefer it medium rare, give it 90 seconds on each side).

Pile up the pasta and top with the sliced cooked tuna and some basil, if using.

★ TOP TIP: MAKE YOUR OWN PESTO

Pesto is one of the most versatile sauces around. It also freezes well – pour into ice cube trays and freeze. I've gone with a classic pesto here, but you can use almost any nut or any cheese that has a strong flavour. A handful of spinach is also a nice touch.

INGREDIENTS

Makes about 300 ml
40g pine nuts
40g parmesan
70g basil, big stalks removed
120ml olive oil
1 clove garlic, roughly chopped

METHOD

Place all the ingredients in a food processor with a pinch of salt and pepper and blitz until smooth.

If you are storing for a few days, pour into an airtight container. It will keep in the fridge for around 4 days.

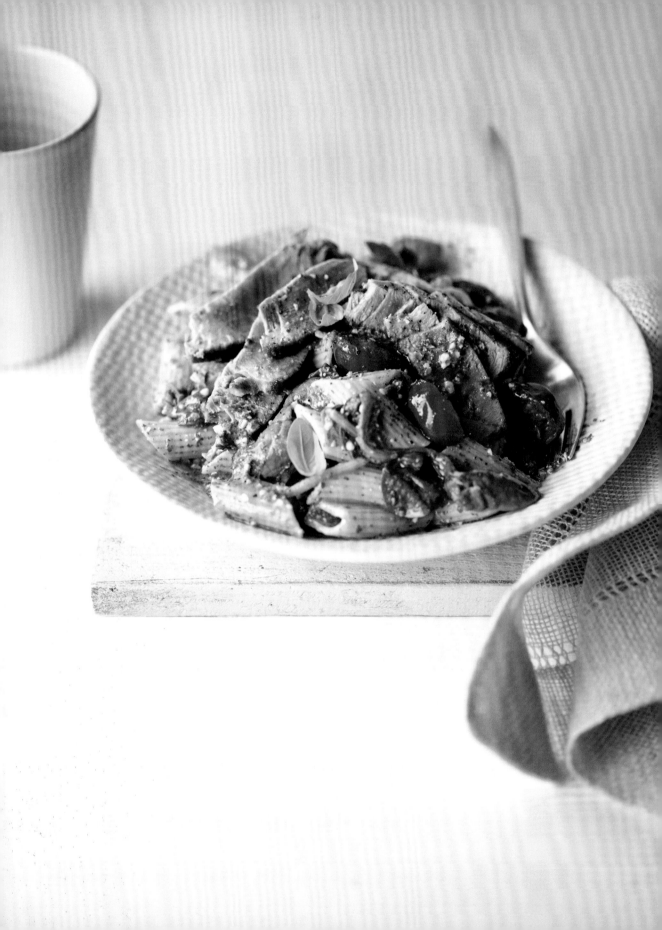

PEPPERED STEAK WITH SWEET POTATO CHIPS

SERVES 1

CARB-RICH
INGREDIENTS

1 large sweet potato
1 tbsp coconut oil
1 tbsp pink peppercorns
1 x 250g sirloin steak, trimmed
  of visible fat
salt
2 tbsp dried breadcrumbs
juice of 1 lemon, to serve

★ Serve with a watercress
side salad.

Steak and chips is such a classic post-workout meal and it never gets old. This peppered one with sweet potato fries is just what you need to get your body building lean muscle.

METHOD

Prick the potato in a few places with a fork and plonk it into your microwave. Zap at 900w for 4 minutes, let it rest for 1 minute then zap for a further 4 minutes.

While the sweet potato is rotating in the microwave, smash up the peppercorns in a pestle and mortar until they are still reasonably big, but there are no whole peppercorns left. Melt half of the coconut oil in a frying pan over a high heat.

Tip the peppercorns onto a plate and coat the steak – they should stick to the meat. Turn the steak until it is fully covered in the peppercorns. Season the steak with a little salt and lay gently into the hot oil. Fry the steak for 3½ minutes on each side before removing to a plate and leaving to rest.

Turn the heat off from under the empty steak pan, and add the dried breadcrumbs. Stir for 1 minute, or until they are crisp. Tip the now delicious crumbs on top of the resting steak.

Take the sweet potato and slice it in half lengthways, then slice each half into 3 wedges to make 6 chunky chips.

Heat the remaining oil in the same frying pan over a high heat and, when melted and hot, carefully slide the sweet potato wedges in and fry for 2–3 minutes, turning a couple of times to brown them evenly. Drain the fried chips on a piece of clean kitchen roll.

Serve up the pretty steak topped with breadcrumbs alongside the sweet potato chips and a side salad of watercress dressed with lemon juice. Perfection.

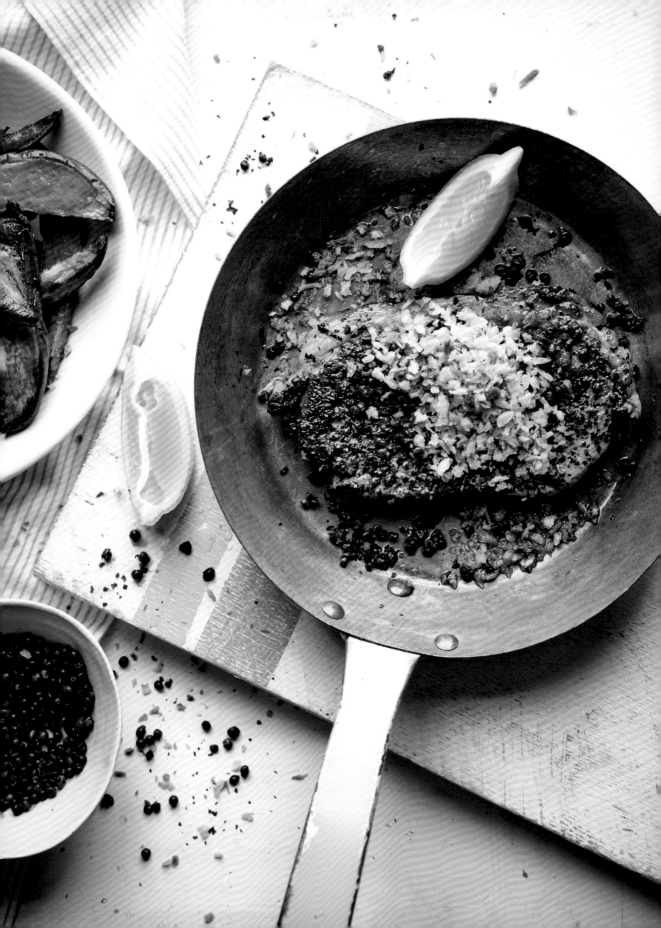

INDONESIAN FRIED RICE

SERVES 1

CARB-RICH
MAKE AHEAD

INGREDIENTS

½ tbsp coconut oil

½ carrot, chopped into 1cm cubes

3 midget trees (tender-stem broccoli), any bigger stalks sliced in half lengthways

¼ red pepper, de-seeded and chopped into 1cm pieces

3 spring onions, finely sliced

2 cloves garlic, chopped

1 x 200g skinless chicken breast fillet, sliced into 1cm thick strips

5 raw king prawns, peeled

250g pre-cooked rice

1 tbsp ketjap manis

1 tsp light soy sauce

1 tbsp chopped coriander

juice of 1 lime, to serve

Just when you thought there were no more ways to fry rice, bam – I've come up with another one. If you don't fancy prawns and chicken then give this a go with beef instead. Ketjap manis is an Indonesian sweet soy sauce, which you can find in most supermarkets.

METHOD

Melt the coconut oil in a large frying pan over a medium to high heat. Add the carrot, midget trees, red pepper, spring onions and garlic and stir-fry for 2 minutes.

Throw in the chicken strips and the prawns, crank up the heat to the max and fry for about 3 minutes, stirring almost constantly. Add the rice, crumbling it between your fingers as you drop it in, and pour in about 2 tablespoons of water.

Continue stir-frying for another 1–2 minutes, breaking up any clumps of rice with a wooden spoon, until the chicken and prawns are cooked through and the rice is hot. Check the chicken is cooked by slicing into one of the larger pieces to make sure the meat is white all the way through, with no raw pink bits left.

Remove the pan from the heat and pour in the ketjap manis and soy sauce.

Serve up a steaming mound of fried rice with the coriander scattered over the top and a squeeze of lime juice.

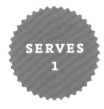

SERVES 1

CARB-RICH
MAKE AHEAD

INGREDIENTS

½ tbsp coconut oil
2 spring onions, finely sliced
1 clove garlic, finely sliced
1 x 240g skinless chicken
   breast fillet, sliced into 1cm
   thick strips
2 sprigs of thyme
5 cherry tomatoes, halved
salt and pepper
big handful of baby spinach
   leaves
180g fresh spaghetti

SPEEDY SPAGHETTI AND CHICKEN

Using fresh spaghetti speeds this one up but if you don't have any you can always use the dried stuff instead. This tastes so good you can eat it cold at lunch too.

METHOD

Bring a large saucepan of water to the boil.

Melt the coconut oil in a frying pan over a high heat. Add the spring onions and garlic and stir-fry for 30 seconds.

Chuck in the chicken and thyme sprigs and continue to stir-fry for 2 minutes until the chicken is almost cooked and starting to brown.

Drop in the cherry tomato halves along with a generous pinch of salt and pepper and reduce the heat to medium. This is a good time to plunge your pasta into the boiling water. Cook the pasta for about 2 minutes (or longer if using dried spaghetti) before draining in a colander.

When the tomatoes have broken down a little, check that the chicken is cooked through by slicing into one of the larger pieces to make sure the meat is white all the way through, with no raw pink bits left. Then add the spinach to the pan and toss with the chicken until wilted.

Remove the pan from the heat and add the cooked spaghetti. Gently toss the ingredients until well combined.

Serve up your super-speedy chicken pasta.

TURKEY MEATBALL AND NOODLE SOUP

SERVES
1

CARB-RICH
MAKE AHEAD

INGREDIENTS

300ml chicken stock
1 lemongrass stalk, white
  part only, sliced in half and
  bashed with the side of
  a knife
1 star anise
4cm ginger, roughly chopped
250g ready-made turkey
  meatballs
4 midget trees (tender-stem
  broccoli), any bigger stalks
  sliced in half lengthways
2 heads of pak choy, sliced in
  half lengthways
200g 'straight to wok' medium
  noodles
1 tbsp fish sauce
juice of 1 lime
1 red chilli, de-seeded and
  finely sliced
1 spring onion, trimmed and
  finely sliced
2 tsp chopped mint
2 tsp chopped coriander

This is one-pot dream cooking, easy to make and with fewer dishes to clean up. This recipe is very loosely based on pho, a Vietnamese noodle dish that lends itself to being personalized, so feel free to add your favourite veg here.

METHOD

Put the kettle on to boil.

Pour the chicken stock into a saucepan and heat until simmering. While the stock is coming to the boil, drop in the bruised lemongrass stalk, star anise and ginger.

When the liquid has come to the boil, drop in the turkey meatballs and let them simmer for about 3 minutes, skimming any froth that appears on the surface.

After 3 minutes, add the midget trees and pak choy and simmer for a further minute.

Remove the noodles from the packet and drop them into a colander. Pour over the water that has boiled in the kettle – this is both to warm the noodles but also to rinse off the weird oil they are coated in – and then shake to cool a little. Carefully pick up the noodles and plop them into the base of a soup bowl.

Check the meatballs are cooked through by cutting into one to make sure there are no raw pink bits left. When you are happy they are done, take the pan from the heat and stir through the fish sauce and lime juice. Pour the hot mixture carefully over the noodles.

Dress the steaming bowl of yumminess with the red chilli, spring onion, mint and coriander.

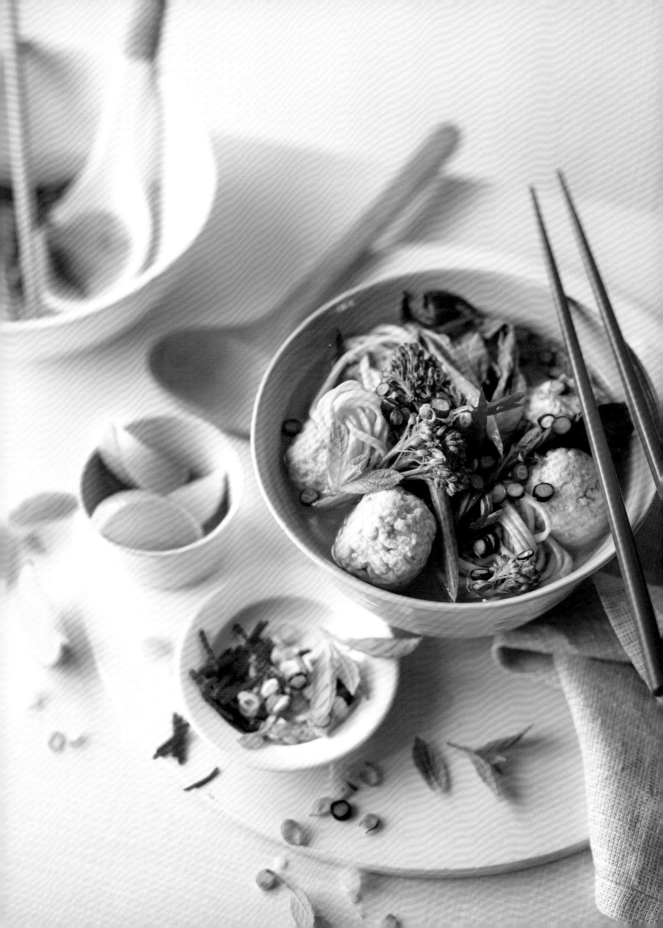

QUICK CHICKEN AND MUSHROOM RISOTTO

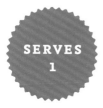

SERVES 1

CARB-RICH INGREDIENTS

100g risotto rice (arborio
  and carnaroli are the most
  common)
½ tbsp coconut oil
¼ leek, finely sliced
5 chestnut mushrooms,
  roughly chopped
1 x 250g skinless chicken
  breast fillet, sliced into 1cm
  strips
salt and pepper
250ml hot chicken stock
2 tbsp chopped parsley
2 tsp chopped chives
juice of 1 lemon, to serve

I used to shy away from risotto, thinking it took too long
and was too much hassle. But then I took a crack at it for
Lean in 15 and came up with this super-tasty shortcut recipe.
I think you'll be surprised how easy this one is and how
great it tastes . . . Enjoy!

METHOD

Bring a saucepan of water to the boil. Drop in your rice and
simmer for 5 minutes before draining through a sieve.

While the rice is cooking, melt the coconut oil in a large
saucepan over a medium to high heat. Add the leek and fry
for 1 minute. Chuck in the mushrooms and chicken strips
and continue to fry for a further 2 minutes, seasoning with
a little salt and pepper.

Throw the drained rice into the saucepan and fry with the
other ingredients for 1 minute. Pour in the hot chicken stock
and bring the liquid up to the boil. Simmer and stir almost
constantly for 5–6 minutes, or until you are sure the chicken
is fully cooked through. To check, slice into one of the larger
pieces to make sure the meat is white all the way through,
with no raw pink bits left.

Remove the pan from the heat and stir through the chopped
herbs. Season to taste and serve up with a squeeze of
lemon juice.

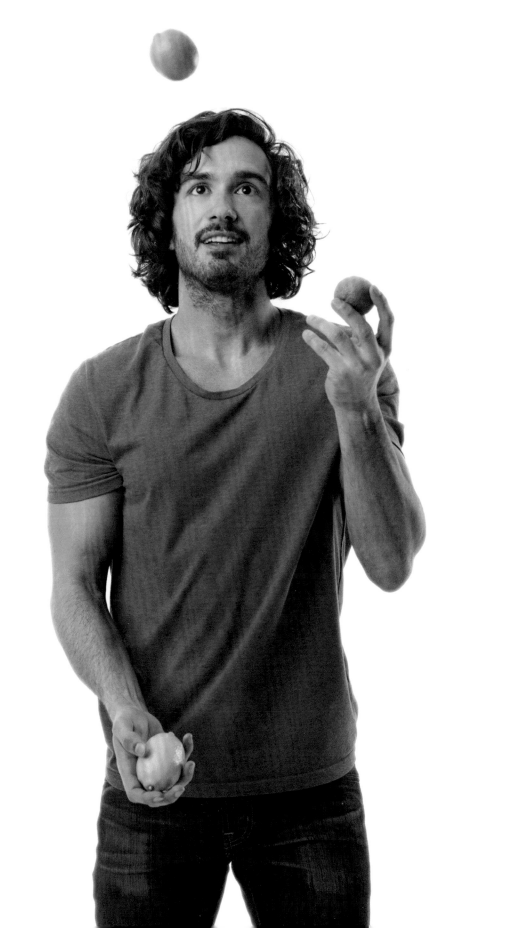

ZAATAR CHICKEN AND CHICKPEA SALAD

SERVES 1

CARB-RICH
MAKE AHEAD

INGREDIENTS

½ tbsp coconut oil

2 spring onions, finely sliced

1 red chilli, finely sliced –
remove the seeds if you
don't like it hot

1 x 200g skinless chicken
breast fillet, sliced into 1cm
thick strips

120g tinned chickpeas,
drained and rinsed

2 tsp zaatar, plus a little extra
for sprinkling

2 tbsp chopped parsley

juice of 1 lemon

salt and pepper

½ cucumber, chopped into
1cm cubes

3 cherry tomatoes, halved

2 tbsp pomegranate seeds

Zaatar sounds like the name of an alien planet but it's actually a really handy spice blend from the Middle East, which is now easy enough to find in most supermarkets. You'll be sprinkling zaatar on everything once you've tried it.

METHOD

Melt the coconut oil in a large frying pan over a medium to high heat. Add the spring onions, red chilli and chicken strips and stir-fry for about 3 minutes, by which time the chicken should be fully cooked through. To check, slice into one of the larger pieces to make sure the meat is white all the way through, with no raw pink bits left.

Tip in the chickpeas and toss together with the chicken for about 1 minute, or until the chickpeas are just warmed through. Take the pan from the heat and add the zaatar, parsley and lemon juice along with a sprinkling of salt and pepper. Toss the whole lot together.

Serve up the chicken and chickpeas topped with the chopped cucumber, tomatoes, pomegranate seeds, and a little extra sprinkling of zaatar.

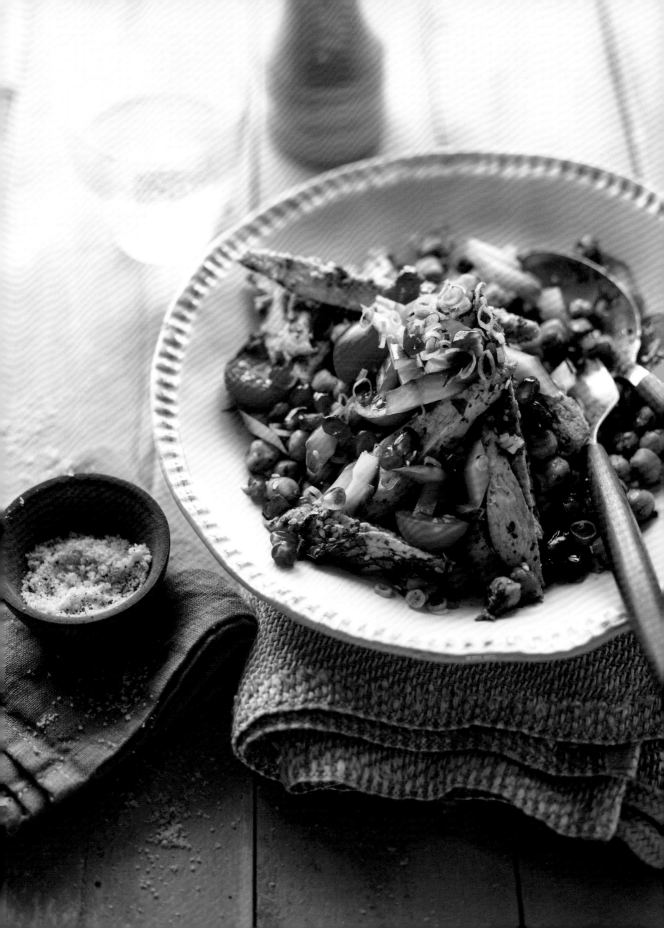

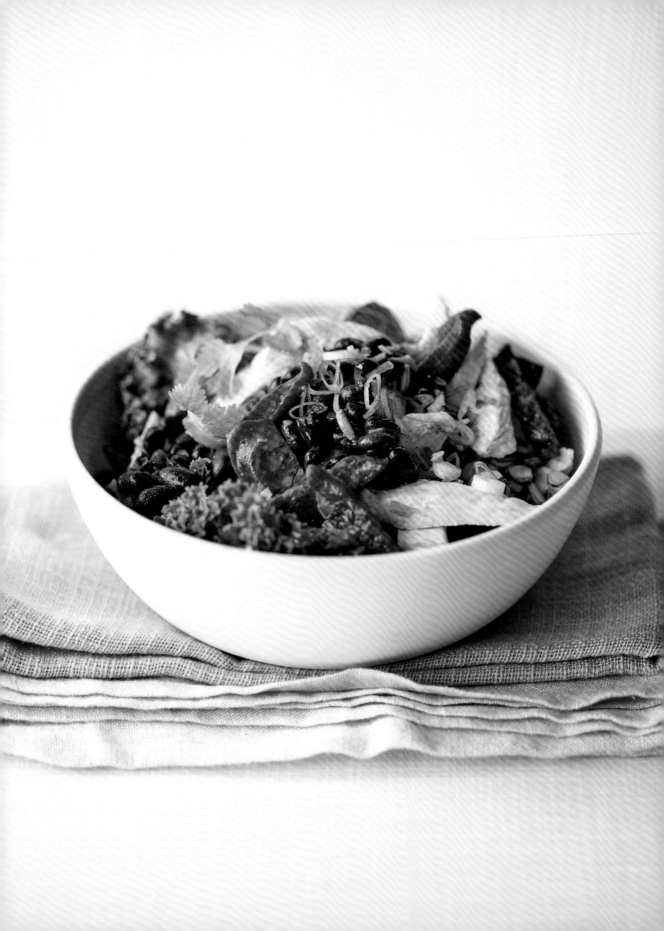

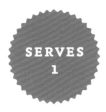

SERVES 1

CARB-RICH
MAKE AHEAD
GOOD TO FREEZE

INGREDIENTS

½ tbsp coconut oil
30g cooking chorizo, chopped
  into 1cm pieces
small bunch of coriander,
  stalks and leaves separated
2 spring onions, finely sliced
1 x 200g skinless chicken
  breast fillet, sliced into 1cm
  thick strips
150g tinned black beans,
  drained and rinsed
75ml chicken stock
juice of 1 orange, to serve

★ Mix in a big portion of
your favourite greens such as
spinach, kale, broccoli, mange
tout or green beans.

BLACK BEANS AND CHORIZO WITH CHICKEN

This is a really hearty and filling post-workout meal. It tastes pretty good cold or reheated the next day too, so is perfect for a lunch box.

METHOD

Melt the coconut oil in a wok or large frying pan over a medium to high heat. Chuck in the chorizo pieces and stir-fry for 1 minute. Roughly chop the coriander stalks and add to the pan along with the spring onions and chicken strips, then stir-fry the whole lot together for 2 minutes.

Tip in the black beans and the chicken stock. Bring to the boil and simmer for 2 minutes, or until you are sure the chicken is fully cooked and the beans are warmed through. Check that the chicken is cooked by slicing into one of the larger pieces to make sure the meat is white all the way through, with no raw pink bits left.

Serve up your dish sprinkled with the chopped coriander leaves and a squeeze of orange juice.

NOODLES WITH STEAK AND MIDGET TREES

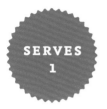

SERVES 1

CARB-RICH
INGREDIENTS

½ tbsp coconut oil

½ red onion, cut into
 6 wedges

2 cloves garlic, roughly sliced

4 midget trees (tender-stem
 broccoli), sliced in half
 lengthways

1 x 240g sirloin steak, sliced
 into 1cm strips

40g mange tout

200g 'straight to wok' medium
 noodles

1 tbsp light soy sauce

2 tsp sesame oil

I'm sure you know by now how much I love a midget tree.
This is a true Lean in 15 dish. Simple, quick and tasty . . . BOSH!

METHOD

Melt the coconut oil in a wok or large frying pan over a high
heat. Add the onion wedges and stir-fry for 1 minute.

Add the garlic and midget trees and stir for a further 45 seconds
before adding in the steak strips and mange tout. Continue to
stir-fry for 2 minutes, by which time the beef will be cooked
medium rare.

Tip in the noodles, breaking up the clumps with your fingers
as you drop them in, along with 2 tablespoons of water, which
will steam up and help the vegetables to cook and the noodles
to separate. Give the whole lot one final minute of stir-frying
until the noodles are warmed through and soft.

Turn the heat off under the pan and pour in the soy sauce and
sesame oil. Toss to dress the stir-fry before piling high on a
plate and diving in with a fork.

CARB-RICH
INGREDIENTS

½ tbsp coconut oil
½ red onion, diced
2 cloves garlic, finely chopped
1 tbsp bhuna curry paste
100g tinned chopped tomatoes
240g raw prawns, peeled
250g pre-cooked basmati rice
large handful of baby spinach
  leaves
2 tbsp chopped coriander
juice of 1 lime, to serve

PROPER PRAWN CURRY

Fancy ordering a takeaway curry? Hold tight. This one will be with you quicker than any geezer on a moped and it's gonna get you lean too.

METHOD

Melt the coconut oil in a wok or large frying pan over a medium to high heat. Add the onion and stir-fry for 2 minutes before chucking in the garlic and continuing to cook for a further minute.

Pour in the curry paste and fry for 1 minute – turn down the heat if it starts to spit at you! Chuck in the chopped tomatoes and stir to combine with the curry paste. Bring the liquid to the boil and simmer for 2 minutes.

Drop in the prawns, bring the liquid back to the boil and simmer for 1–2 minutes, or until the prawns have turned pink, which indicates they are fully cooked.

Ping your rice in the microwave according to the packet instructions.

Stir the spinach and coriander through the prawns, and cook just long enough for the spinach to wilt into the liquid.

Serve up the rice topped with the curry and a squeeze of lime juice.

SERVES 1

CARB-RICH
MAKE AHEAD

INGREDIENTS

1½ tbsp tomato ketchup
2 tsp harissa paste
1 large or 2 small pittas
shredded iceberg lettuce
4 cherry tomatoes, halved
¼ cucumber, sliced into
  half-moons
100g deli-style cooked ham
  (not the processed stuff)
150g deli-style cooked chicken,
  shredded
2 pickled green chillies, to
  serve
1 gherkin, to serve

FULLY LOADED CHICKEN PITTA

A bit like the famous build-up bagel from Book 1, this is a recipe that you'll be smashing more than once a week. #Guilteeeeee.

METHOD

Mix together the ketchup and harissa paste until smooth and fully combined.

Zap the pitta bread(s) in the microwave for 10 seconds at 900w. When warm, slice about 1cm from the long side of the pitta, which should make it easy to prise it open.

From now on it's up to you to freestyle, but this is how I build mine: spread about half of the spicy ketchup on the base of the warm pitta and stuff a good amount of shredded lettuce into the bottom along with a few bits of tomato and cucumber. Now stuff the ham and chicken into the pitta and then top with any remaining lettuce, tomatoes and cucumber.

Drizzle the remaining sauce all over and serve with the pickled green chillies and sliced gherkin.

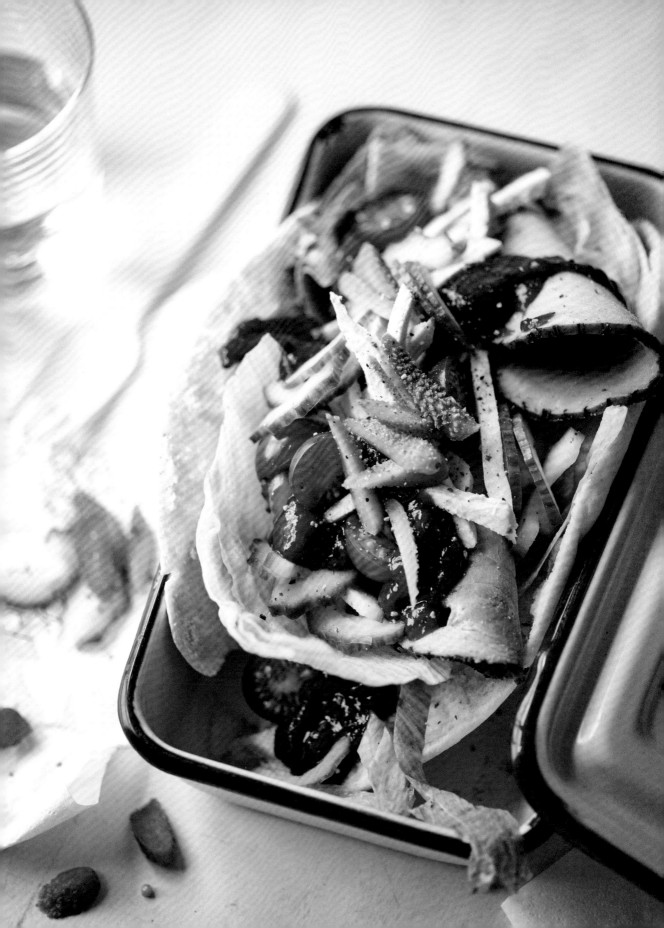

THE BODY COACH HOTDOGS

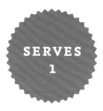

**SERVES
1**

CARB-RICH
INGREDIENTS

2 rashers of smoked back
  bacon, chopped into thin
  strips
180g turkey mince
1 egg
20g fresh breadcrumbs
¼ tsp ground mace
pinch of white pepper
½ tsp ground coriander
salt
2 large hotdog rolls
French mustard, to serve
ketchup, to serve

★ Serve alongside a big bowl
of green salad.

Everyone knows hotdog sausages are full of rubbish so I wanted
to create a healthy and lean version, and I think I've absolutely
nailed it with this one. They look a bit odd but, trust me, they
taste incredible and feel like a real treat after a workout.

METHOD

Preheat your grill to maximum.

Drop the bacon strips into a food processor along with the
turkey mince, egg, fresh breadcrumbs, ground mace, white
pepper and ground coriander. Add a good pinch of salt and
blitz the ingredients until they become a smooth mix – this
is best done using the pulse function.

Tip the mixture into a small bowl and, using damp hands, take
a quarter of the mix at a time and roll into rough sausage shapes.
Place them on a baking tray lined with baking parchment and
slide them under the grill for 10 minutes, turning regularly.

Before you eat the hotdogs, check they are fully cooked through
by cutting into one to make sure the meat is white all the way
through, with no raw pink bits left.

Serve up two big dogs in each roll, top with mustard and
ketchup, and get it down you.

CARB-RICH
MAKE AHEAD
GOOD TO FREEZE
(the ragu, not the
potatoes)

INGREDIENTS

150g baby new potatoes,
   biggest ones chopped in half
½ tbsp coconut oil
½ red onion, diced
1 celery stick, diced
¼ courgette, diced
2 sprigs of thyme
1 x 240g sirloin steak, sliced
   into 2cm thick strips
2 tsp tomato puree
2 tsp sherry, balsamic or red
   wine vinegar
100g tinned chopped tomatoes
salt and pepper
chopped parsley, to serve –
   optional

QUICK BEEF RAGU WITH NEW POTATOES

Ragu is normally the result of hours of bubbling away – well not in my book: this is ready in 15 minutes. I'm not afraid to shout, 'WALLOP!' as I throw the potatoes in the microwave either.

METHOD

Place the potatoes in a microwaveable bowl and add a splash of boiling water. Cover with cling film and zap in the microwave at 900w for 3 minutes. Rest the potatoes for 1 minute and then zap for a further 3 minutes. Leave them in the microwave until you are ready to eat.

Melt the coconut oil in a large frying pan over a medium to high heat. Add the onion, celery, courgette and thyme sprigs and stir-fry for 2 minutes.

Crank up the heat to maximum, drop in the steak strips and fry for 1 minute. Squeeze in the tomato puree and stir in, followed swiftly by the vinegar which should quickly bubble away to almost nothing.

Pour in the chopped tomatoes and bring up to the boil before reducing the heat to a simmer. Season with salt and pepper and stir through the chopped parsley, if using.

Serve up the spuds topped with the speedy ragu and chow down.

CARB-RICH
MAKE AHEAD

INGREDIENTS

1 tbsp coconut oil

3 spring onions, finely sliced

1 celery stick, chopped

½ dessert apple, peeled and
   roughly chopped

1 tbsp chopped coriander

2 tsp curry powder

salt and pepper

100ml chicken or vegetable
   stock

1 x 240g skinless chicken
   breast fillet

75g fresh breadcrumbs

1 egg white

200g pre-cooked rice

1 red chilli, sliced, to serve –
   optional

CHEEKY CHICKEN KATSU

This is a banger and one of my favourite meals to make.
If you've got some mates coming round, knock this up and
they'll be well impressed.

METHOD

Melt half of the coconut oil in a saucepan over a medium heat.
Add the spring onions, celery, apple and coriander and fry for
1 minute. Throw in the curry powder and a good pinch of salt
and continue to stir-fry for 45 seconds. Pour in the stock and
bring to the boil before simmering for 10 minutes.

While the sauce is cooking, place the chicken breast between
two pieces of cling film, or even better two pieces of baking
parchment, on a chopping board. Using a rolling pin, saucepan
or any other blunt instrument, bash the breast until it is about
1.5cm thick all over – this is a decent workout. Slide the beaten
chicken to one side.

Next, pour the breadcrumbs into a bowl. Whisk up the egg
white until it is a little frothy, then dip the flattened chicken
into the egg and then straight into the breadcrumbs. Push the
crumbs into the chicken so that as many stick to it as possible.

Melt the remaining coconut oil in a frying pan over a medium
to high heat and cook the chicken for 3 minutes on each side,
by which time it should be fully cooked through – check by
slicing into the thickest part to make sure the meat is white
all the way through, with no raw pink bits left. This is a good
time to zap your rice in the microwave according to the
packet instructions.

When your sauce has simmered for 10 minutes, blitz the
ingredients using a blender until smooth. Taste and season
with a little more salt and pepper if needed.

Slice the chicken and serve up with the rice topped with the
yummy sauce and, if using, a sprinkling of fiery red chilli slices.

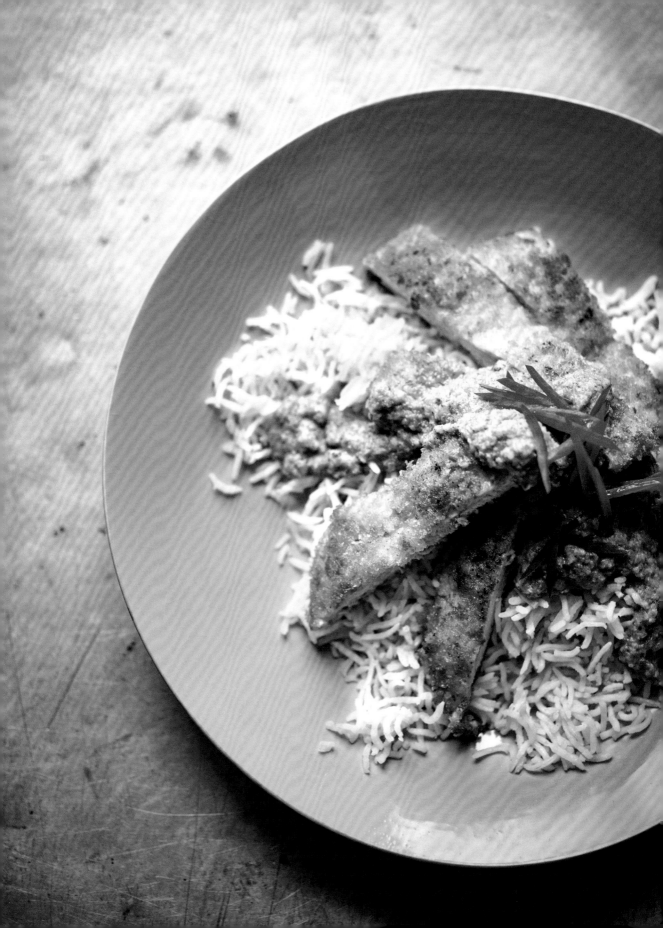

HOT AND SOUR BEEF NOODLES

CARB-RICH
MAKE AHEAD

INGREDIENTS

½ tbsp coconut oil

½ red pepper, de-seeded and finely sliced

1 clove garlic, chopped

2cm ginger, chopped

3 spring onions, finely sliced

1 x 240g sirloin steak, sliced into 1.5cm thick strips

salt and pepper

3 midget trees (tender-stem broccoli), any bigger stalks sliced in half lengthways

40g mange tout or green beans

250g 'straight to wok' noodles

2 tsp honey

1 tbsp red wine vinegar

2 tsp light soy sauce

2 tsp sesame oil

chopped coriander, to serve

This is a dish to blow away the cobwebs, a full-on flavour assault. It's another one that keeps well in a lunch box and can be thrown in the microwave and eaten at work.

METHOD

Melt the coconut oil in a wok or large frying pan over a medium to high heat. Add the red pepper, garlic, ginger and spring onions. Stir-fry together for 1 minute.

Add the steak strips and continue to stir-fry for 1 minute, adding a little salt and pepper. Toss in the midget trees, mange tout and noodles, breaking up the clumps as you drop them in, and continue to stir-fry for 30 seconds. Pour in 2 tablespoons of water and let it steam up through the ingredients, helping to cook the veg and to warm the noodles through.

Drizzle in the honey then immediately pour in the red wine vinegar, which will bubble up in a cloud. Continue to stir-fry for about 1 more minute, by which time everything should be hot.

Remove the pan from the heat and mix in the soy sauce and sesame oil. Sprinkle with chopped coriander and serve up straight away to appreciate the kick.

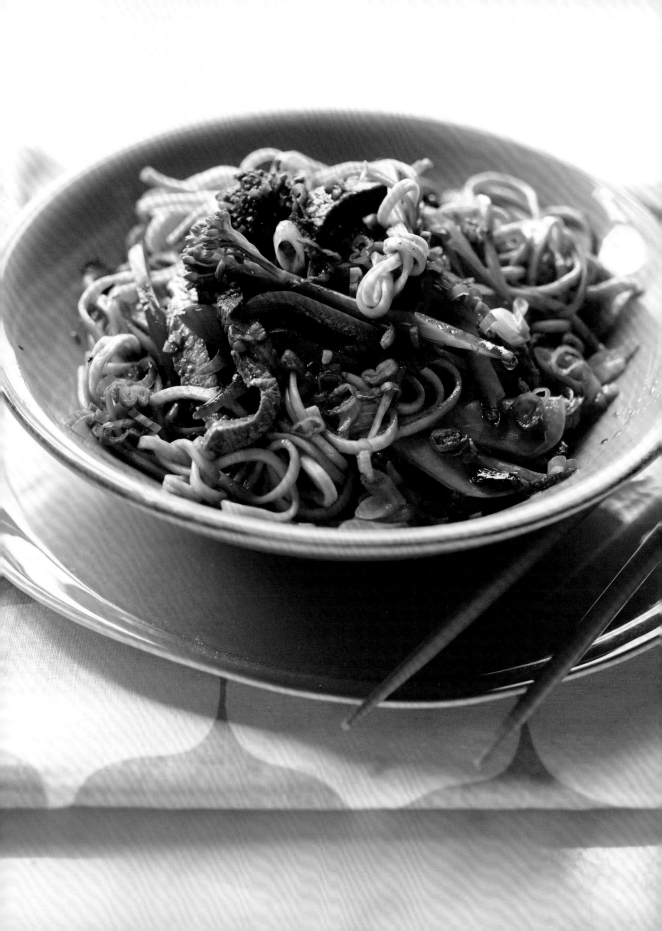

PRAWN AND CHILLI TAGLIATELLE

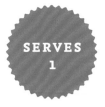

SERVES 1

CARB-RICH
INGREDIENTS

75g dried tagliatelle
3 midget trees (tender-stem
  broccoli), any bigger stalks
  sliced in half lengthways
½ tbsp coconut oil
3 spring onions, finely sliced
½ tsp dried chilli flakes
4 cherry tomatoes, halved
1 clove garlic, chopped
240g raw king prawns, peeled
salt and pepper
juice of 1 lemon

A classic combination. Sweet prawns and hot chillies are
a match made in heaven. Cooking the vegetables in the
same pan as the pasta saves time and washing up – win, win.
As you can see, I've doubled the recipe in the picture.

METHOD

Bring a large saucepan of water to the boil. When boiling,
add the tagliatelle and cook for 12 minutes, or according to the
packet instructions. About 2 minutes before the cooking time
is up, drop the midget trees into the same pan and continue
to cook. Drain the pasta and trees together in a colander.

While the pasta is cooking, melt the coconut oil in a frying
pan over a medium to high heat. Add the spring onions, chilli
flakes, tomatoes and garlic and stir-fry for 1–2 minutes, or
until the tomatoes are starting to soften.

Tumble in the prawns and stir-fry the whole lot together for
2 minutes, or until the prawns have changed to a deep pink,
which indicates they are fully cooked.

When you're happy the prawns are cooked, turn off the heat
and tip the pasta and midget trees into the frying pan. Toss the
whole lot together, adding a good pinch of salt and pepper.

Pile the pasta high on your plate, squeeze over some lemon
juice and chow down.

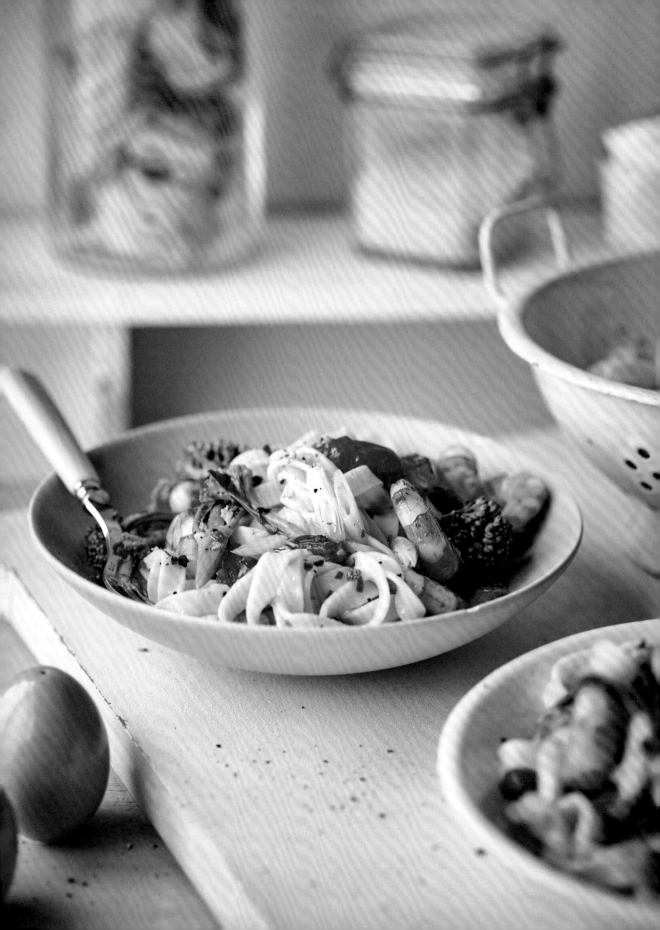

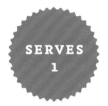

CARB-RICH
LONGER RECIPE
INGREDIENTS

1 medium baking potato
  (about 225g)
1 chicken sausage
1 large tomato, halved
salt and pepper
2 rashers of turkey bacon
2 tbsp plain flour
3 eggs
½ tbsp coconut oil
large handful of baby spinach
  leaves

THE BODY COACH FRY-UP

I do like to pop down to the cafe for a fry-up sometimes but it's not always cooked the healthiest way. Here's my version of a fry-up, which will sort you out the Body Coach way and curb your cravings for a greasy full English. This recipe should take you around 25 minutes.

METHOD

Preheat your grill to maximum and put a saucepan of water on to boil.

Prick your potato with a fork in four or five places and put it in the microwave. Zap at 900w for 4 minutes, let it rest for 3 minutes, turn it over and zap for a further 4 minutes. Leave to cool.

Meanwhile, lay the sausage on a baking tray and slide it under the grill. Cook for 3–4 minutes before turning. Sprinkle the tomato halves with a little salt and pepper and slide under the grill with the sausage for 3 minutes. Lay the bacon on the same tray and cook everything together, turning as necessary, until it is all fully cooked through. Shut the door and turn the grill off to keep everything warm until you're ready to eat.

When the potato is cool enough to handle, cut it open and scoop the flesh from the skin into a bowl. Add the flour to the potato, crack in an egg and add a generous pinch of salt and pepper. Beat the ingredients together until you have a stiff mixture. Using clean hands, form two large potato cakes from the mix.

Melt the coconut oil in a large frying pan and slide in the potato cakes. Fry on each side for about 2 minutes, or until nicely browned.

Crack open the remaining 2 eggs into the boiling water, reducing the heat until the water is just 'burping'. Poach them for 4–5 minutes, or until the white has set but yolk is still runny, then carefully lift out with a slotted spoon and drain on paper towels.

When the potato cakes are cooked, remove them from the pan and throw the spinach into the still-hot pan to wilt.

Serve up the sausage, bacon and tomato alongside the potato cakes and spinach, then top it off with the poached eggs – life is good.

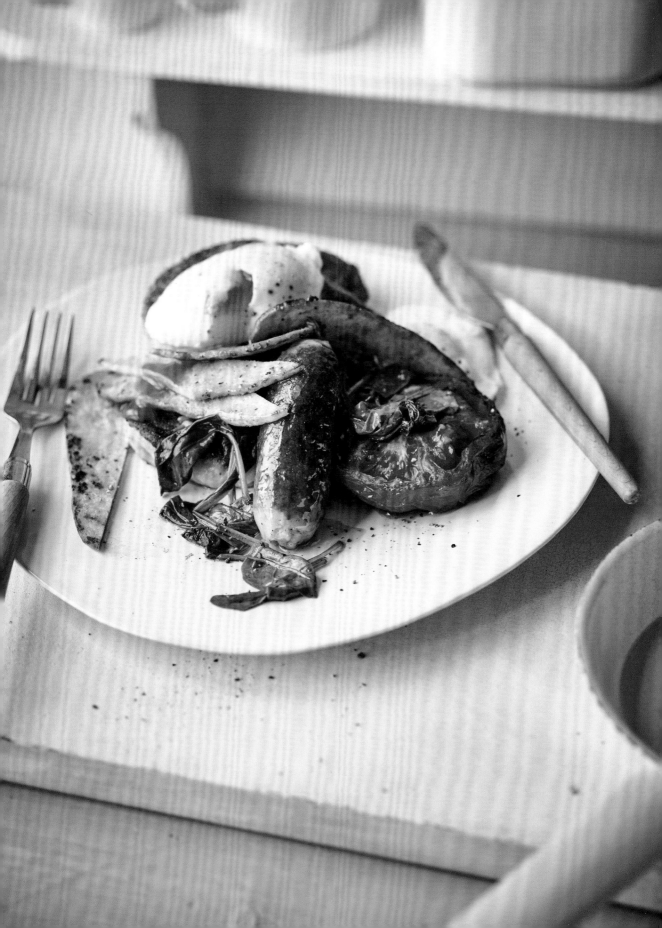

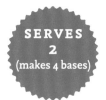

CARB-RICH
GOOD TO FREEZE
(the bases, not the topping)
LONGER RECIPE
INGREDIENTS

350g plain flour, plus a little
   extra for dusting
75g full-fat Greek yoghurt
150ml warm water
salt and pepper
1–2 tbsp coconut oil
150ml passata
200g beef mince
1 tbsp dried Italian herbs
1 x 250g skinless chicken
   breast fillet, sliced into thin
   strips
150g cooked ham, sliced into
   thin strips
1 green pepper, de-seeded and
   sliced into thin strips
handful of black olives, halved
a few basil leaves

★ Serve with a large green
side salad.

SLOPPY JOE'S PIZZA

This is a cheat's base for a pizza which, once cooked, can be
frozen and then cooked from frozen with fresh toppings.
It should take you 45 minutes and is a really fun recipe to make
with your kids, so if you've got any little ones, get them involved.

METHOD

Preheat your oven to 190°C (fan 170°C, gas mark 5).

Tip the flour into a bowl and add the yoghurt and warm water
along with a good pinch of salt. Get your hands in and mix
together, tipping it out onto a floured surface and kneading until
you have a smooth dough. Shape into a ball, drop into a clean
bowl, cover with cling film and leave to rest for 15 minutes.

After the dough has rested, roughly divide it into 4. Roll out
each portion to the size of a dinner plate, about 1.5cm thick.

Melt a little of the coconut oil in a large non-stick frying pan
over a medium to high heat. Carefully lay one dough portion
into the hot oil and fry for 90 seconds on each side. Remove
the cooked base and repeat with the remaining dough, adding
a little more oil as necessary. If you're just eating one serving
then this is the time to freeze the other bases for another day.

Pour the passata into a bowl and add the beef mince, Italian
herbs and a good pinch of salt and pepper. Mix together until
well combined. Spread the beef and tomato mix over the bases –
Sloppy Joe style – and then scatter the chicken, ham, pepper
and olives evenly over the pizzas.

If you have a normal-sized oven then you will probably only be
able to bake two pizzas at a time. Bake each pizza for 25 minutes,
or until you are sure all the meat is fully cooked through, with
no raw pink bits left.

Scatter the cooked pizza with basil leaves, slice up and serve.
Bellissima!

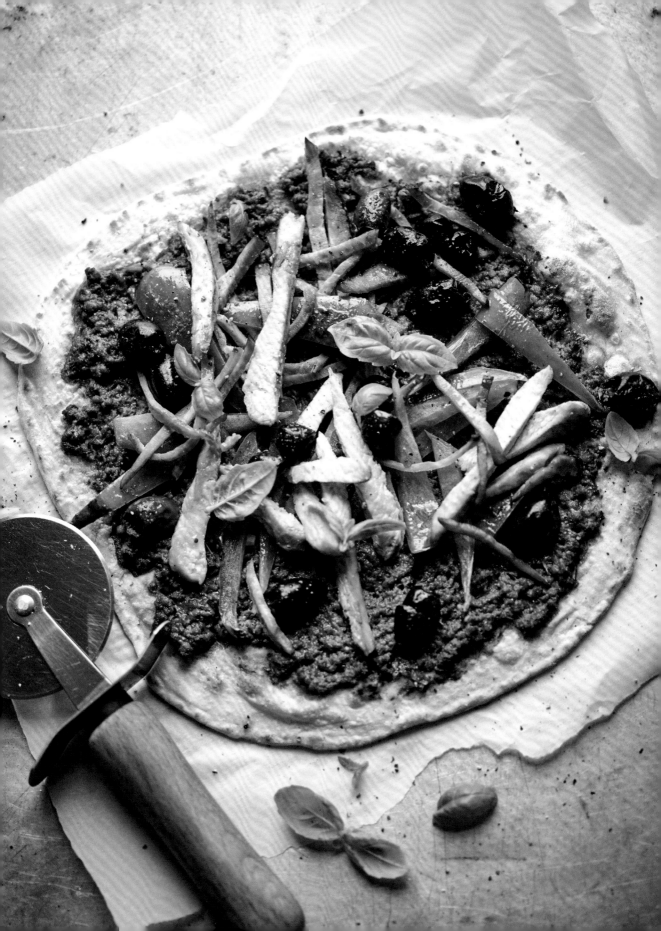

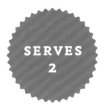

SERVES 2

CARB-RICH
MAKE AHEAD
LONGER RECIPE
INGREDIENTS

½ butternut squash
few drizzles of olive oil
salt and pepper
7 sage leaves
5 midget trees (tender-stem
   broccoli), any bigger stalks
   sliced in half lengthways
130g quinoa, uncooked weight
¼ cucumber, sliced into 1cm
   pieces
6 radishes, sliced
500g cooked skinless chicken
   breast, sliced
juice of 2 lemons
small handful of alfalfa
   sprouts (pea shoots or
   mustard cress would work
   very well too)
3 tbsp pomegranate seeds

BUTTERNUT, CHICKEN AND QUINOA SALAD

Sometimes people just stick a load of ingredients that are good for you in a salad, but they forget the flavour. Not me – this is *all* about the flavour. It takes longer than 15 minutes (more like 50 minutes) but it's a great one to batch-cook for a couple of days' time.

METHOD

Preheat your oven to 190°C (fan 170°C, gas mark 5) and bring a large saucepan of water to the boil.

Prepare your squash by peeling it, discarding the seeds, and then roughly chopping the flesh into 2cm chunks. Place the chunks on a roasting tray, then drizzle with olive oil and sprinkle with a little salt and pepper before sliding into the oven and roasting for 10 minutes.

After 10 minutes, remove the squash from the oven, add the sage and the midget trees to the roasting tray and toss to mix. Continue to roast the ingredients for a further 10 minutes, by which time the squash and trees should be cooked and a little golden in places. Remove and leave to cool.

While the vegetables are roasting, cook the quinoa in plenty of boiling salted water according to the packet instructions. When it is cooked, drain in a sieve, rinse under cold running water and tip into a large bowl. Add the cucumber, radishes, chicken, lemon juice, a drizzle of olive oil and a pinch of salt and pepper. Mix the whole lot together.

When the squash and midget trees have cooled to room temperature, mix them through the quinoa, and then pile your plates high with the delicious salad. Finish with a crown of alfalfa sprouts and a scattering of pomegranate seeds.

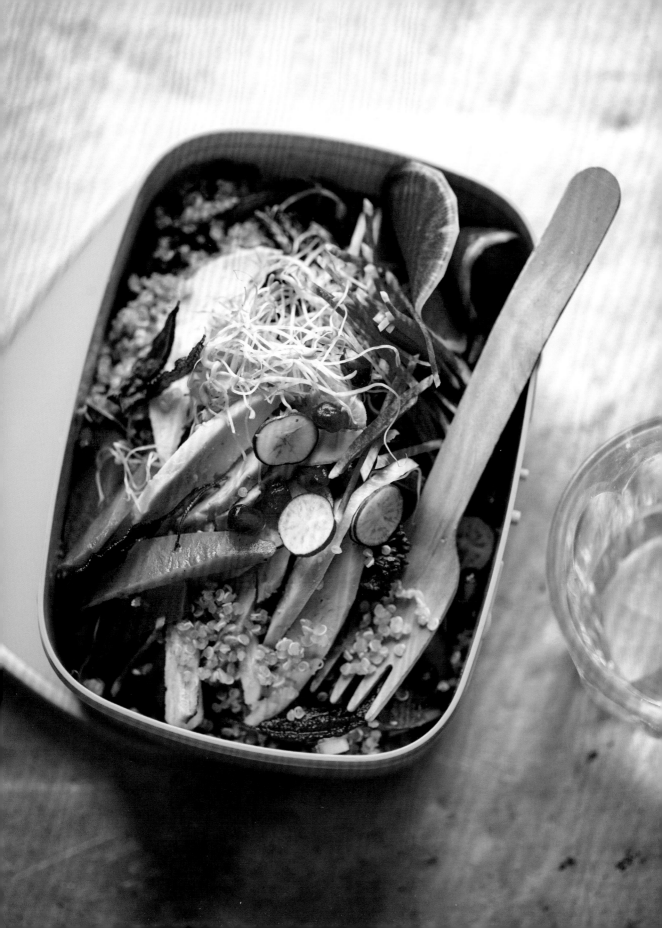

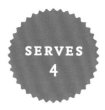

CARB-RICH
MAKE AHEAD
LONGER RECIPE
INGREDIENTS

2 tbsp coconut oil

2 small onions, diced

4 cardamom pods, lightly crushed

5 cloves

1 large cinnamon stick, snapped in half

2 bay leaves

5 cloves garlic, chopped

5cm ginger, chopped

1 green chilli, finely chopped – remove the seeds if you don't like it hot

1 tbsp garam masala

1kg boneless and skinless chicken thighs, sliced into bite-sized pieces

500g cauliflower florets, large florets cut in half

350g basmati rice

1 x 400g tin of chopped tomatoes

450ml chicken stock

5 tbsp chopped coriander

5 tbsp pomegranate seeds

CHICKEN AND CAULIFLOWER BIRYANI

This is the first time in this book that I'm using chicken thighs but as it's a longer recipe (it should take you 50 minutes in total) there is time for them to cook through and it's going to taste so much better than using breast. This is a beast of a meal, so pick your largest casserole dish and get cooking.

METHOD

Melt the coconut oil in a large flameproof casserole dish over a medium to low heat. Throw in the onions, cardamom pods, cloves, cinnamon and bay leaves. Fry the ingredients, stirring regularly, for 5–6 minutes, or until the onions are just soft.

Add the garlic, ginger and chilli to the pot and continue to stir for a further 2 minutes.

Sprinkle in the garam masala and fry, stirring almost constantly, for 45 seconds. Increase the heat to maximum and add the chicken pieces and cauliflower florets. Fry the ingredients together for 1 minute – if you feel the spice is burning the base of the pan then just pour in a splash of water.

Add the rice, the chopped tomatoes and the chicken stock to the pot and bring to the boil. Give the biryani one last stir, place a lid on top and reduce the heat to very low. Leave to cook for 20 minutes before turning off the heat completely and leaving to stand for 5 minutes.

Just before serving, rough up the rice with a fork and garnish with chopped coriander and pomegranate seeds.

CARB-RICH
MAKE AHEAD
GOOD TO FREEZE
LONGER RECIPE
INGREDIENTS

150g dried red lentils
1½ tbsp coconut oil
1 large red onion, diced
2 cinnamon sticks
5 cardamom pods, bashed
  with the side of your knife
4 cloves garlic, chopped
5cm ginger, chopped
2 red chillies, finely sliced –
  remove the seeds if you don't
  like it hot
1½ tbsp garam masala
2 tsp ground ginger
1 x 400g tin of chopped
  tomatoes
300ml chicken stock (from a
  cube is fine)
480g skinless chicken breast
  fillet, cut into large 5cm
  chunks
salt and pepper
5 tbsp chopped coriander
juice of 2 limes, to serve

CHICKEN AND LENTIL CURRY

This is another recipe that needs a bit more love and attention, so it takes a little more time than my usual Lean in 15 meals – 50 minutes plus 1 hour soaking time. It's well worth the effort, though, and you can cook the curry up in a big batch and freeze it for the week ahead.

METHOD

Tip the lentils into a bowl, cover with plenty of cold water and leave to soak for 1 hour. After 1 hour, drain the lentils in a sieve, then rinse under cold running water.

Melt the coconut oil in a large saucepan over a medium to high heat. Add the onion, cinnamon and cardamom pods and fry, stirring regularly, for 4 minutes before scraping in the garlic, ginger and chillies.

Fry for 2 minutes, then sprinkle in the garam masala and ground ginger and fry, stirring constantly, for 30 seconds. Chuck in the drained lentils and pour in the chopped tomatoes and chicken stock. Bring the whole lot to the boil and simmer for about 30–35 minutes, by which time the lentils should be nice and soft.

Add the chunks of chicken and simmer for a further 10 minutes, or until you are sure the chicken is fully cooked – check by cutting into a thick piece to make sure the meat is white all the way through, with no raw pink bits left.

Finally, add in the salt, pepper and coriander. Serve up the delicious lentils with a final squeeze of lime juice.

LOADED POTATO SKINS

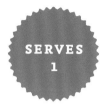

CARB-RICH
LONGER RECIPE
INGREDIENTS

1 large baking potato
  (about 275g)
20g ricotta
1 spring onion, finely sliced
1 tbsp chopped parsley, plus a
  little extra for sprinkling
150g cooked skinless chicken
  breast
75g cooked deli-style ham
1 egg
black pepper

★ Serve with a green side salad.

These are naughty. And I don't mean bad. I mean good. Really good. Is there anything better than a baked potato loaded with chicken and ham? Oi, mate, don't forget to prick your spud with a fork before zapping it in the microwave – if not you'll blow the door off. This one will take you 40 minutes.

METHOD

Prick the potato in at least 4 places with a fork. Place in the microwave and zap at 900w for 4 minutes. Leave to rest for 4 minutes, then flip over and zap for a further 4 minutes. Leave the potato to rest until cool enough to handle.

Preheat your oven to 200°C (fan 180°C, gas mark 6).

When you are able to handle the spud, slice it in half and carefully scoop the cooked flesh from the inside into a bowl. Add the ricotta, spring onion, chopped parsley, chicken, ham and egg to the potato along with a grind of fresh black pepper. Beat the ingredients together until they're well mixed.

Spoon the mix back into the potato skins – you will find that they will be overflowing a little. Place the filled skins on a baking tray and slide into the oven.

Bake for 10–12 minutes, or until the top of the filling is nicely browned.

Remove, serve up with the remaining parsley and a simple salad, and drift off to a happy place.

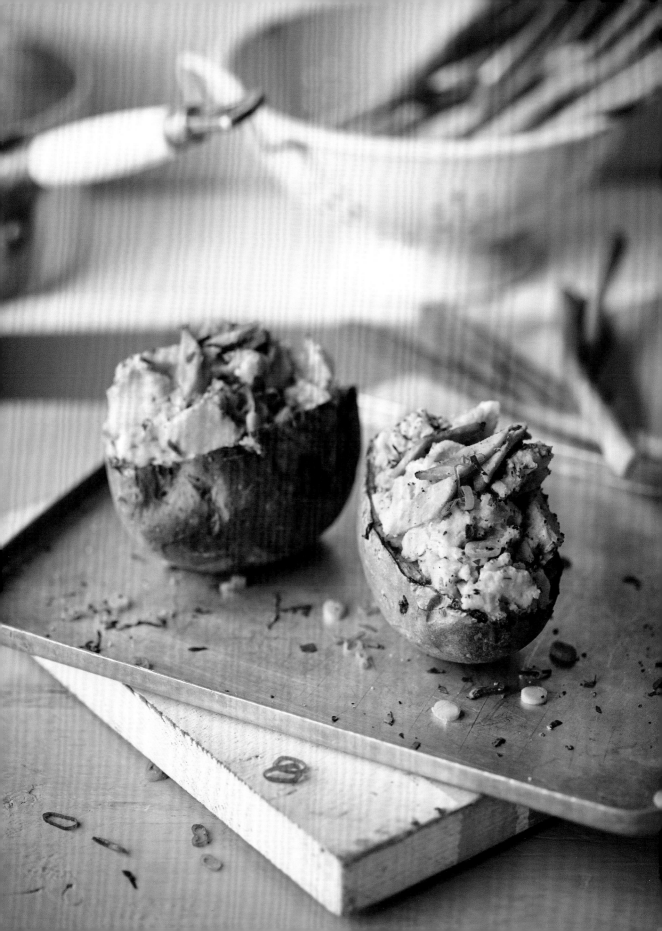

CARB-RICH
MAKE AHEAD
LONGER RECIPE
INGREDIENTS

600ml chicken stock (from
  a cube is fine)
pinch of saffron strands
1 tbsp coconut oil
1 red onion, roughly diced
1 cinnamon stick, snapped in
  half
2 tsp cumin seeds
600g stewing lamb, leg or
  neck is best, cut into 2–3cm
  chunks
3 cloves garlic, roughly diced
2 ripe tomatoes, roughly
  chopped
80g dried apricots, cut in half
200g tinned chickpeas,
  drained and rinsed
100g couscous
4 tbsp chopped coriander, to
  serve

LAMB TAGINE

This takes the same time as a football match to cook
(90 minutes) so prep it, whack it in the oven and kick back
with a coldie until you hear the alarm go off. Make sure
you check on it and give it a good old stir at half-time.

METHOD

Heat up 400ml of the chicken stock and, when warm, add
the saffron strands. Leave to steep and get on with the rest
of the recipe.

Melt the coconut oil in a large flameproof casserole dish over
a medium to high heat. Add the onion, cinnamon and cumin
seeds. Fry the ingredients for 2 minutes, by which time the
onion should be softened.

Crank up the heat to maximum and add the lamb chunks and
garlic to the dish. Stir-fry the ingredients for 2–3 minutes.
Add the chopped tomatoes, dried apricots and saffron-infused
chicken stock. Bring the whole lot to a simmer and cook for
about 1 hour 15 minutes, or until the meat is soft and tender.

When there is about 15 minutes of cooking left, add the
chickpeas to the tagine and let them warm through.

Place the couscous in a bowl. Bring the remaining 200ml
of chicken stock to the boil in a saucepan and pour over the
couscous. Cling-film the bowl and let the couscous sit for
10 minutes.

Serve up the tagine with the couscous, all topped with an
artistic scattering of chopped coriander.

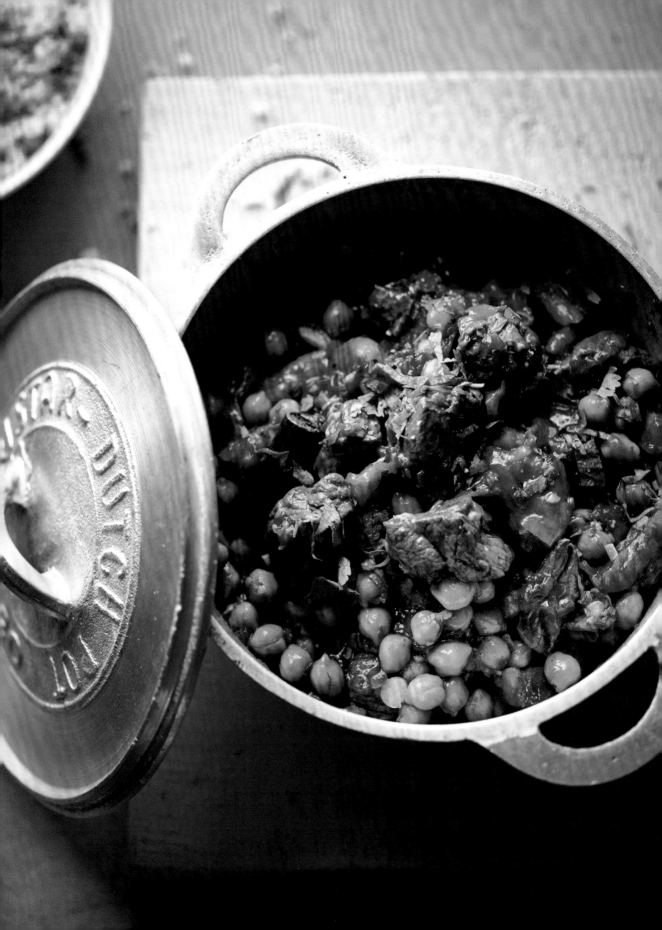

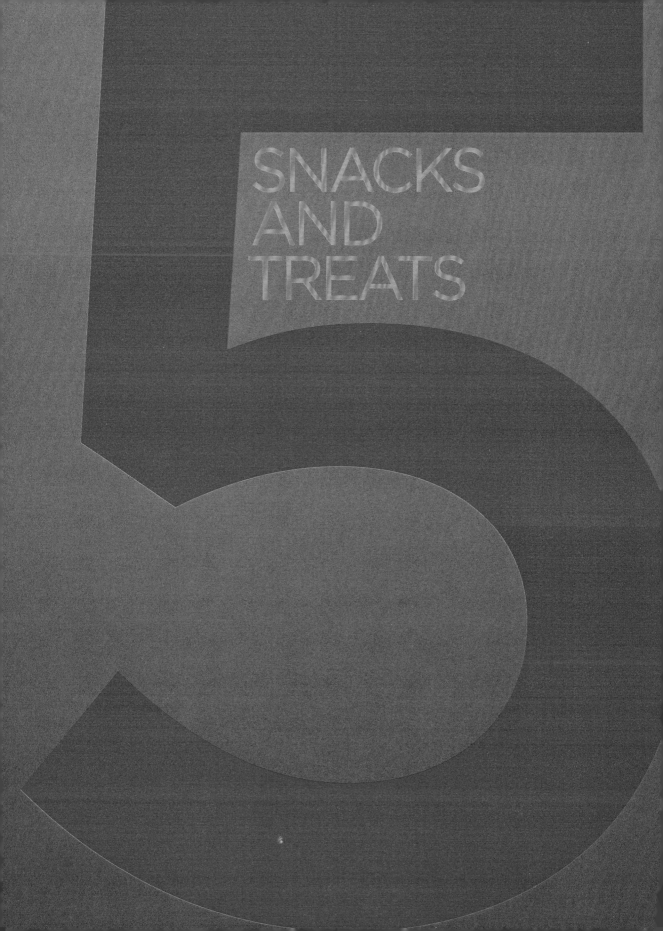

SNACKS AND TREATS

5

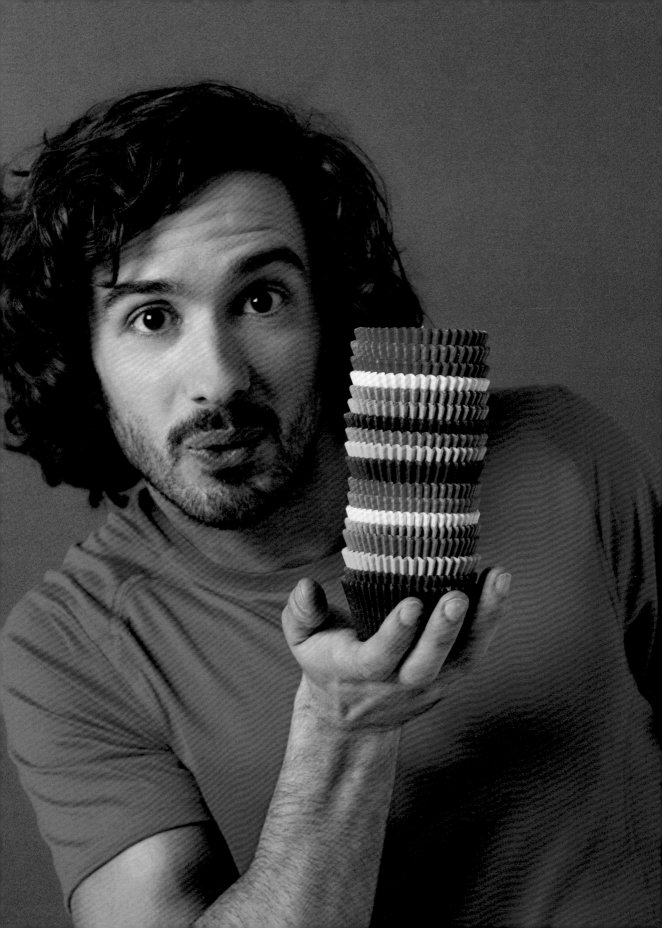

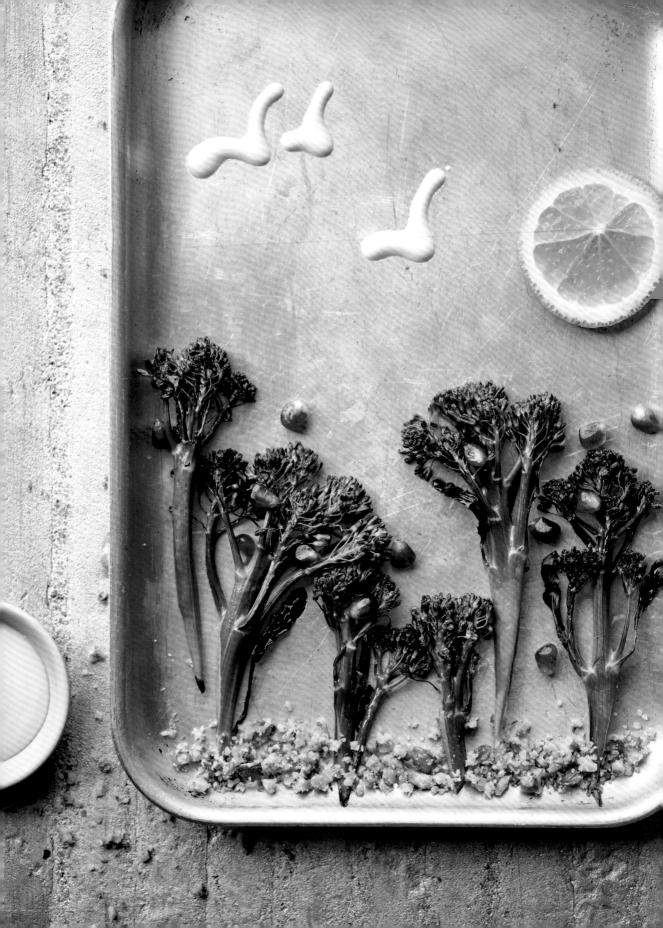

ROASTED MIDGET TREES WITH TAHINI

SERVES 1

Everybody else is banging on about roasting kale and parsnips; well, I'm roasting midget trees. This makes such a great little snack. Don't forget to shout, 'Oooh, midget trees!' as you throw them in the oven.

INGREDIENTS

1 tbsp coconut oil

200g midget trees (tender-stem broccoli), any bigger stalks sliced in half lengthways

1 red chilli, finely sliced – remove the seeds if you don't like it hot

salt

1 tbsp tahini

1 tbsp full-fat Greek yoghurt

juice of 1 lemon

1 tbsp extra virgin olive oil

1 tbsp pomegranate seeds – optional

METHOD

Preheat your oven to 220°C (fan 200°C, gas mark 7).

Dollop the coconut oil onto a roasting tray, then scatter over the midget trees along with the chilli and a good pinch of salt. Roast the trees in the oven for 14 minutes, turning halfway through.

While the trees are roasting, mix together the tahini, yoghurt, lemon juice, olive oil, a pinch of salt and 2 tablespoons of warm water until you have a smooth sauce.

When the midget trees have had their time, remove them from the oven and either leave to cool a little or tuck straight in. I like to plate them up – sometimes I like to get creative and make them look like little trees! – pour over the sauce and then top with pomegranate seeds.

★ TOP TIP

Haven't heard of tahini? It's a protein-rich paste made from ground sesame seeds – mix 1 tablespoon of the stuff with a splash of water, 1 chopped garlic clove and a squeeze of lemon juice for a tasty salad dressing!

SMOKED SALMON AND BUTTER BEAN DIP

SERVES 1

MAKE AHEAD

INGREDIENTS

100g tinned butter beans
  (drained weight)
black pepper
1 small clove garlic, roughly
  chopped
100g smoked salmon, roughly
  chopped
50g cream cheese
1 tbsp chopped chives
1 tbsp chopped parsley
juice of 1 lemon
sprinkling of nigella seeds –
  optional
1 ripe avocado, sliced, to serve
vegetable batons, to serve

Butter beans may be unfashionable, but they're good for you and taste great so let's give them a chance and bring 'em back. The dip will keep in an airtight container in the fridge for up to 3 days.

METHOD

Put the kettle on to boil. Tip the butter beans into a bowl and pour over enough boiling water to cover. Leave the beans to soak for 5 minutes.

When the beans have had their 5 minutes, drain them in a sieve and put in a small food processor along with 2 tablespoons of water and a generous grind of pepper. Add the garlic, smoked salmon, cream cheese, chopped herbs and lemon juice and blitz the ingredients until you have a thick puree.

Serve up the dip topped with nigella seeds, if using, alongside slices of avocado and vegetable batons.

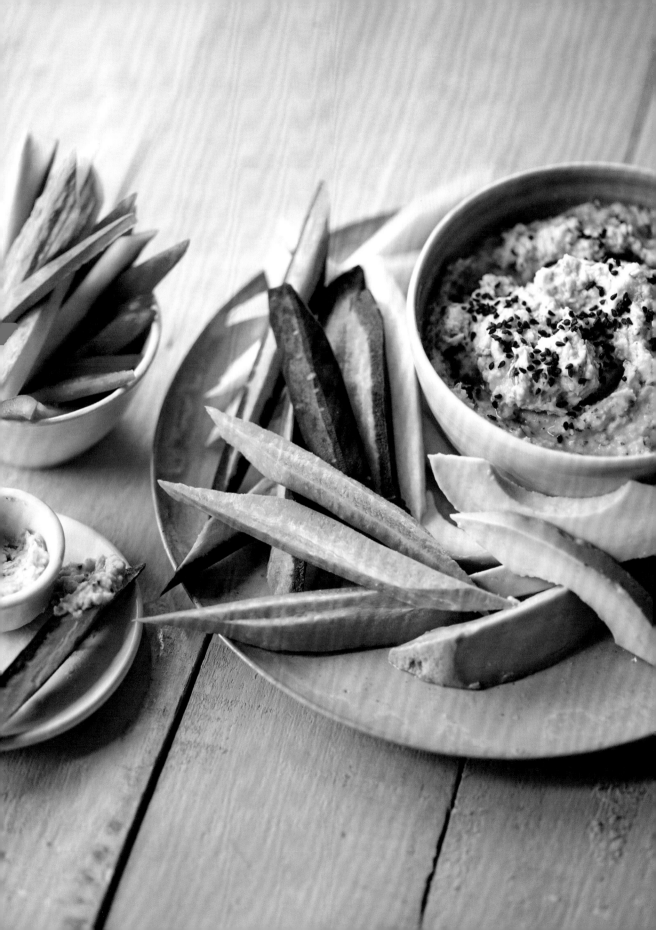

WHIPPED BEETROOT AND FETA

SERVES 1

MAKE AHEAD
INGREDIENTS

2 cooked beetroots, roughly
  chopped
2 tbsp cream cheese
40g walnuts, roughly chopped
40g feta
2 tbsp chopped chives, plus a
  few extra for garnish – optional
salt and pepper
raw vegetable batons, to serve
sprinkling of nigella seeds,
  to serve – optional

Beetroot and feta are besties in this recipe. They work so well together. It makes an awesome snack for dipping carrots and cucumber batons in, or spread on rice cakes.

METHOD

Place all the ingredients, apart from the vegetable batons, into a food processor along with a splash of warm water and a generous pinch of salt and pepper, and blitz until just smooth.

Your dip is ready to serve immediately so sprinkle on the extra chives and nigella seeds, if using, or it can be stored in the fridge for up to 3 days.

THE WORLD'S BEST GUACAMOLE

SERVES 1

MAKE AHEAD
INGREDIENTS

juice of 3 limes
½ red onion, finely diced
2 ripe avocados
1 red chilli, de-seeded and finely
  chopped, plus extra to serve
½ bunch of coriander, leaves
  only, finely chopped, plus
  extra to serve
2 tsp toasted sesame seeds
salt and pepper

Slightly overripe avocados are perfect for this recipe and it will keep in an airtight container in the fridge for 3 days. I soak the red onions in the lime juice to reduce their oniony-ness, which is a major win if you plan to kiss anyone later on.

METHOD

Pour the juice of 2 of the limes into a bowl and add the diced onion. Leave to marinate for 10 minutes.

Meanwhile, cut the avocados in half and de-stone them, then scoop the flesh out into large chunks and put into a bowl. Add the chilli, coriander, sesame seeds, a generous pinch of salt and pepper and the juice of the last lime.

Drain the soaked onion in a sieve and add to the bowl. Use the back of a fork to 'smash' the ingredients together until they form a well-combined mix. Serve with some extra chilli and coriander, if you like.

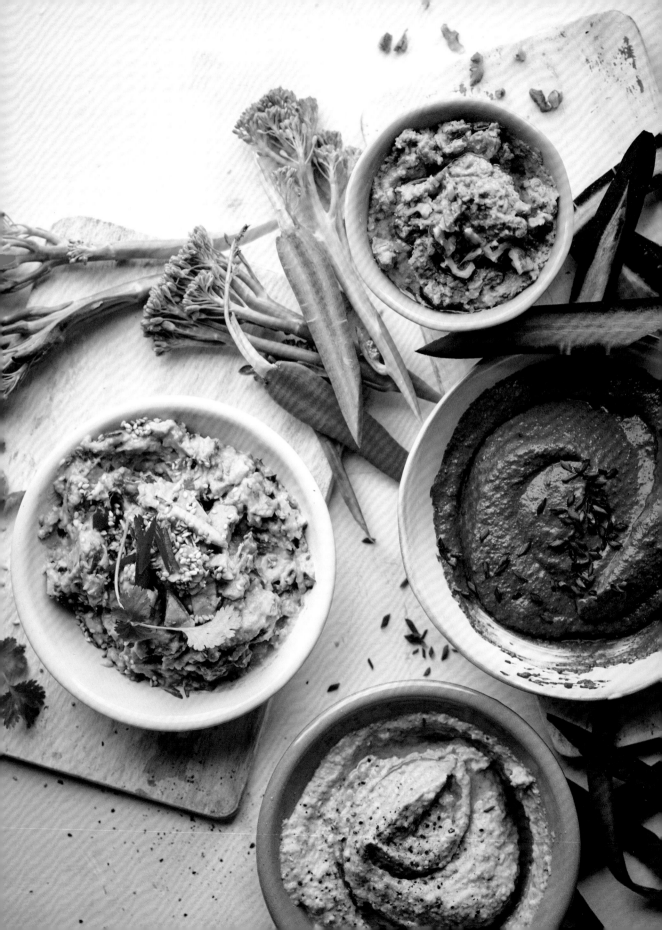

WALNUT WHIP HUMMUS

SERVES 1

Making a homemade hummus is the nuts. This walnut one tastes wicked and will keep in your fridge in an airtight container for up to 4 days.

MAKE AHEAD
INGREDIENTS

150g walnuts
1 x 400g tin of chickpeas, drained and rinsed
1 small clove garlic, roughly chopped
1 tbsp tahini
juice of 1–2 lemons
drizzle of extra virgin olive oil
salt and pepper
sprinkle of cayenne – optional
carrot, cucumber and celery batons, to serve

METHOD

Bring a kettle to the boil. Tip the walnuts into a bowl and cover with boiling water. Leave them to sit for 5 minutes.

Tip the chickpeas, garlic, tahini, the juice of 1 lemon and a drizzle of olive oil into a food processor. Add the walnuts and 2 tablespoons of the soaking water to the ingredients in the processor. Sprinkle in a generous pinch of salt and pepper and blitz together until they reach a smooth consistency.

Taste the hummus and add more salt, pepper or lemon juice if you feel it needs it. Just before serving with the raw vegetables, sprinkle with a little cayenne for an Eighties-inspired presentation.

ALMOND BUTTER BABA GHANOUSH

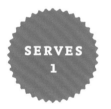

SERVES 1

This takes 17 minutes to make but once you've made it you won't look back. It keeps in the fridge for 3 days. It's great, not only as a dip but also as an accompaniment to fish or meat for a reduced-carb meal.

MAKE AHEAD
LONGER RECIPE
INGREDIENTS

2 aubergines
1 clove garlic, halved
1 tbsp almond butter
juice of 1 lemon
drizzle of olive oil
salt and pepper
raw vegetable batons, to serve

METHOD

Preheat your grill to maximum.

Cut a deep slit into the side of each aubergine and stuff a garlic clove half into each slit. Place the aubergines onto the grill pan or a baking tray and slide under your grill, close to the heat. Grill for 12 minutes, turning a couple of times – don't worry about the skin burning.

After 12 minutes, remove the cooked aubergines from the grill, and when cool enough to handle, slice in half, scoop out the flesh and chuck it into a food processor.

Add the almond butter, lemon juice and olive oil along with a generous pinch of salt and pepper and then blitz until virtually smooth. Your baba ghanoush is now ready for your veg.

PRAWN AND SWEETCORN FRITTERS

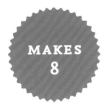

MAKES 8

MAKE AHEAD
GOOD TO FREEZE
INGREDIENTS

250g raw prawns, peeled
3 spring onions, roughly
  chopped
½ courgette, roughly chopped
1 red chilli, roughly chopped –
  remove the seeds if you
  don't like it hot
2 tbsp chopped coriander
100g tinned creamed
  sweetcorn
1 egg yolk
1 tbsp cornflour
salt and pepper
1 tbsp coconut oil
light soy sauce, to serve

Snacks can be a bit boring but these are decent. They freeze well too, so make a big batch while you're at it. After they're cooked, place on a lined baking tray and freeze. Once frozen they can be stacked up. To reheat, just place in a hot oven for 10 minutes.

METHOD

Place all the ingredients apart from the coconut oil and soy sauce into a food processor along with a good pinch of salt and pepper, and pulse until they are well mixed but haven't been turned to mush.

You will probably have to cook the fritters in two batches, unless you have a super-sized frying pan, so melt half of the coconut oil in a large non-stick frying pan over a medium to high heat. When the pan is hot, dollop in 4 large dessertspoons of the mix, spreading them a little with the back of your spoon.

Fry the fritters for about 2 minutes on each side. The raw grey colour of the prawns should turn to glorious pink, which shows you they are cooked.

When you are happy they are cooked, slide them out of the pan and drain any excess oil on a clean piece of kitchen roll. Repeat the process with the remaining coconut oil and mixture until you have 8 delicious fritters.

Serve the fritters warm or at room temperature with a little soy sauce.

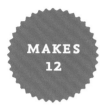

MAKE AHEAD
INGREDIENTS

8 pitted dates, Medjool if
possible
100g ground almonds
2 tbsp flaxseeds
2 tbsp chia seeds
2 tbsp sunflower seeds
2 tbsp cacao nibs
4 tbsp unsweetened
desiccated coconut

ENERGY BALLS

I'm not going to pretend these are a miracle snack that
you can scoff every day and burn fat. They're a treat, so make
a batch and spread them out over a few days or share them
with your friends at work.

METHOD

Bring a kettle of water to the boil and then pour enough water
over the dates to fully immerse them. Leave to sit and soften
for 5 minutes.

When the dates have had their 5-minute bath, thoroughly drain
them in a sieve and blitz in a small food processor with
2 tablespoons of warm water (use the soaking water if you like).
Tip the pureed dates into a bowl and pour in the remaining
ingredients, apart from the coconut.

Mix the ingredients until they become a stiff gloop. Using wet
hands, roll the mixture into 12 golf ball-sized rounds.

Finally, roll the balls in the desiccated coconut.

These balls of energy will keep in an airtight container lined
with baking parchment in a cool, dark place for up to 4 days.

INGREDIENTS

½ avocado, de-stoned and
peeled
175ml coconut water
75g raspberries
15g chia seeds

COCO-BERRY SMOOTHIE

Here's a lovely little smoothie packed with healthy fats to give
you an energy boost.

METHOD

Place all the ingredients into a blender and blitz until smooth.

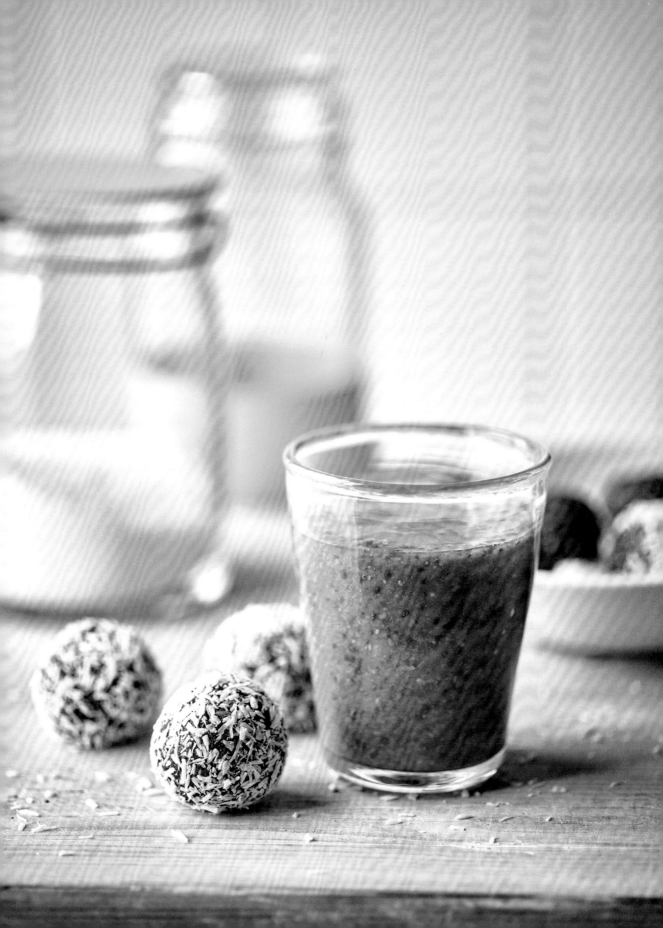

THE VEG PATCH JUICE

SERVES 1

If you're not a fan of eating veg in your main meals then this is a good way for you to get your greens in. Remember, though, a juice is a snack alongside a meal, not a replacement for a meal. The body needs more energy than that, so fuel it.

INGREDIENTS

2 cooked beetroots

2 carrots

large handful of spinach

2 apples

2cm ginger

1 scoop (30g) strawberry
protein powder

METHOD

Pass all the ingredients apart from the protein powder through a juicer. Thoroughly whisk the powder into the juice.

Neck.

★ TOP TIP
SNACK IDEAS

If you don't have time to make a snack, here are a few ideas for you!

- ★ Scoop of whey protein with water
- ★ 20–30g nuts
- ★ 85g beef jerky
- ★ Boiled egg
- ★ 75–100g fruit (melon, blueberries, strawberries, raspberries, apple or pear)

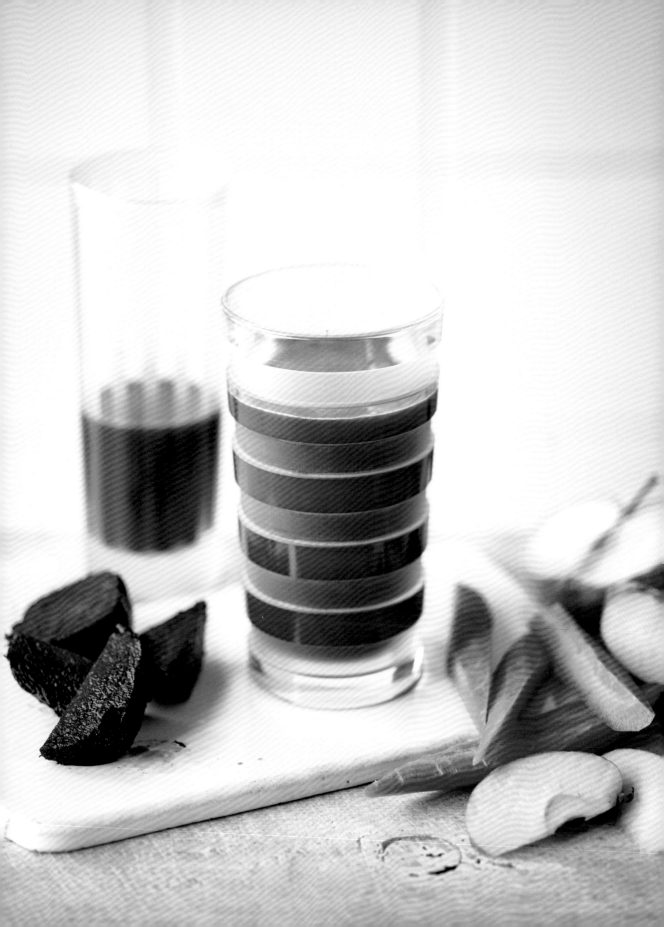

MAKE AHEAD
LONGER RECIPE
(quick to make but needs
4 hours in the freezer)

INGREDIENTS

1 banana, chopped into 2cm
  chunks
150g ripe raspberries
splash of almond milk
1 scoop (30g) vanilla protein
  powder
1 tsp vanilla extract
1 tbsp almond butter
toasted pecans, to serve

DAIRY-FREE RASPBERRY ICE CREAM

This is for those days when you're really craving something sweet. It's a nice little treat to have but serves two, so be sure to make it with a friend or you'll end up eating the lot and falling asleep on the sofa.

METHOD

Spread the fruit over a tray lined with baking parchment, ensuring everything is well spaced. Slide into the freezer and leave to freeze overnight, or for a minimum of 4 hours.

When ready to eat your ice cream, remove the frozen fruit from the freezer and leave to warm up for 5 minutes.

Place the fruit in a food processor along with all the other ingredients apart from the pecans. Pulse the ingredients until they reach a thick ice cream consistency.

Serve up scoops of the ice cream topped with the toasted pecans.

PEANUT BUTTER PROTEIN COOKIES

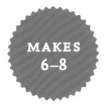

MAKES 6–8

MAKE AHEAD

INGREDIENTS

60g smooth peanut butter
1 scoop (30g) chocolate
   protein powder
1 tsp vanilla extract
30g ground almonds
1 egg
¼ tsp bicarbonate of soda

Did someone say cookies? Guilteeeee. I turned into a cookie monster when I made these for the first time and smashed the lot in about 20 minutes, so be careful!

METHOD

Preheat your oven to 180°C (fan 160°C, gas mark 4) and line a baking tray with baking parchment.

Put all the ingredients in a bowl and beat them with a wooden spoon until smooth. Dollop out mounded tablespoons of the mixture (about the size and shape of a Ferrero Rocher) onto the baking tray, leaving a gap of about 5cm between the mounds.

Bake the cookies for 5 minutes, then remove from the tray and leave to cool on a wire rack (see picture overleaf).

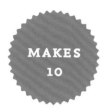

MAKE AHEAD
LONGER RECIPE
INGREDIENTS

2 medium carrots, grated
  (130g)
2 medium eating apples,
  peeled and grated (170g)
100g ground almonds
60g raisins
1½ tsp mixed spice
1 tsp ground cinnamon
1 tsp baking powder
75g ricotta
3 eggs
2 tsp vanilla extract
125g cream cheese
2 tsp honey

CARROT AND APPLE MUFFINS

These are a great little snack to eat with a cup of tea.
I mean, who doesn't love a muffin? They'll take 40 minutes
to make so why not invite some friends over and enjoy
them together?

METHOD

Preheat your oven to 180°C (fan 160°C, gas mark 4) and line
a 12-hole muffin tin with small muffin cases.

Place all the ingredients apart from 1 teaspoon of the vanilla
extract, the cream cheese and the honey in a large bowl and
beat with a wooden spoon until fully combined.

Divide the mixture equally among the muffin cases and slide
into the oven. Bake the muffins for 25 minutes, by which time
they will be cooked through and a little golden on the top.
Leave to cool.

While the muffins are cooling, whip together the remaining
vanilla extract, cream cheese and honey, adding a splash of
water to slacken if needed.

When the muffins are totally cool, spread the cream cheese
icing on top.

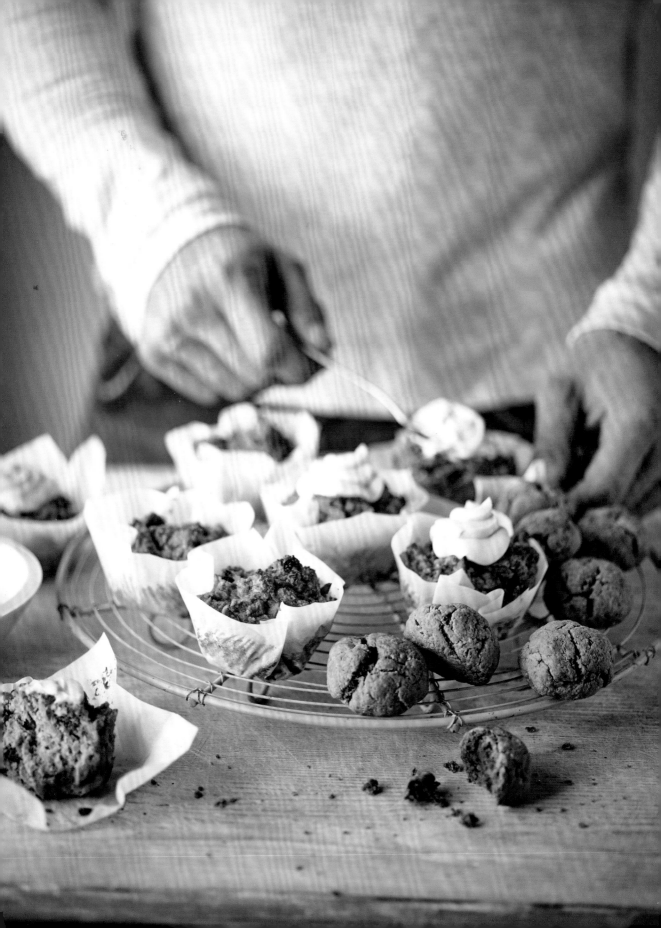

6

VOLUME
RESISTANCE
HIIT
TRAINING

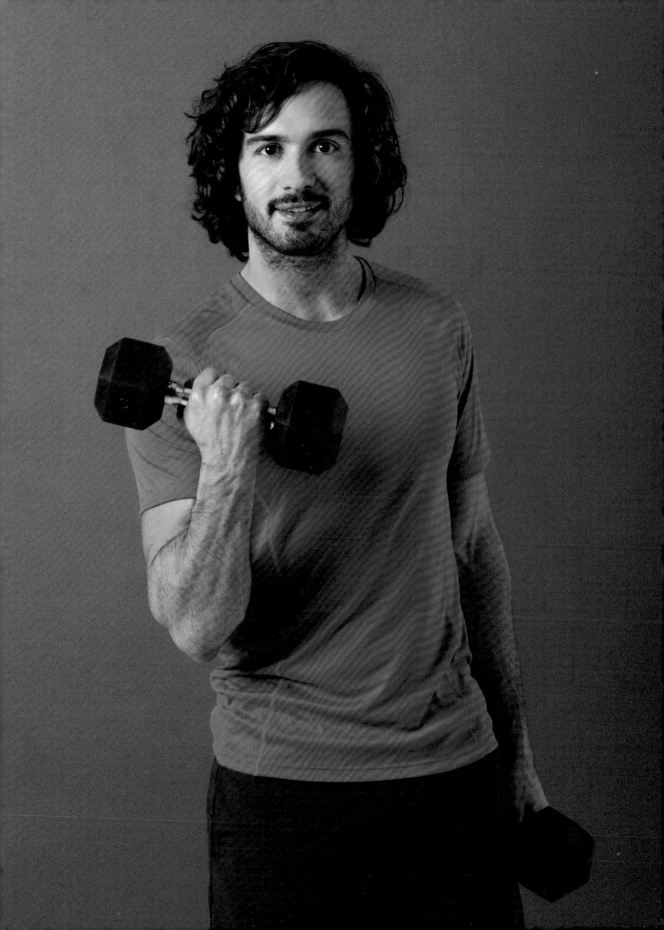

This cycle is all about building lean muscle while reducing body fat. Remember, if you increase your lean body mass, you increase your resting metabolic rate. And this is a good thing because it means you burn more fat and get to enjoy even more food each day, #Win.

I'm now introducing a new form of training I like to call Volume Resistance HIIT, where you combine two rounds of high intensity cardio with two rounds of weight training. This routine not only allows you to build muscle and get strong, it also rapidly improves your cardio fitness levels. It's something all my online clients aim to do four days per week. To say this method is effective for fat loss and lean muscle gain is an understatement and the results my clients get meant I just had to include it in this book.

The effect of the routine on metabolic rate is insane – it will get ramped up, so your body will be burning more and more calories post-workout and at rest.

The great thing about the training plan is that it can be done at home with minimal equipment, so you don't need an expensive gym membership. It's also suitable for people of all fitness levels as you get to choose the weights you lift and the type of cardio exercises you perform based on your own fitness. Always check with your doctor first before starting a new exercise regime if you have any health concerns.

As you get stronger and make more progress, you can increase the weights and intensity.

WHAT IS VOLUME RESISTANCE HIIT?

You may or may not be familiar with a training method called German Volume Training (GVT). It's extremely effective for building lean muscle. It sounds scary but it's really not. It basically involves choosing an exercise (e.g. a bench press) and picking a weight that allows you to complete 10 sets consisting of 10 repetitions per set (100 reps in total) with a 1-minute rest between each set.

I've taken this traditional GVT method and squashed it between two rounds of HIIT cardio, hence the name 'Volume Resistance HIIT'. Just in case you're not familiar with HIIT, here's a quick recap.

WHAT IS HIIT CARDIO?

HIIT cardio means high intensity interval training and involves short bursts of intense maximal effort followed by a resting or recovery period. You can apply it to any cardio machine or body weight exercise such as running on the spot, burpees or mountain climbers. Let's take a treadmill, for example. You will sprint for

20–30 seconds at maximum effort, then walk or jog to recover for 30–45 seconds. You then repeat this several times. The aim of HIIT is to elevate your heart rate to near-maximum during the short working sets, so choose exercises that challenge you. You don't have to do the same type of HIIT all the time either. That can get boring so mix it up. You could do outdoor hill sprints one day, then use the cross-trainer or rowing machine another day.

This type of training is extremely effective for burning fat as it creates what's known as an after-burn effect. It means you not only burn calories during the workout but you also burn calories for hours post-workout. It's hard work at the time but it's over quickly and it makes you feel like an absolute winner afterwards.

HOW OFTEN WILL I TRAIN?

You will aim to do four sessions per week with three full rest days. There are four workouts detailed in this chapter, which focus on a different muscle group each time:

1. Arms
2. Chest and back
3. Legs
4. Shoulders

Each session is to be performed only once a week. You can spread your workouts across your week to suit you but I recommend doing no more than two training days in a row before taking a rest day. These rest days are essential for muscle growth and recovery and will enhance your results, so enjoy them. Be sure to do all four of the workouts during the week to get a total body workout.

Here is how my ideal training week looks:

Monday – CHEST AND BACK
Tuesday – ARMS
Wednesday – REST
Thursday – LEGS
Friday – REST
Saturday – SHOULDERS
Sunday – REST

Remember, you can train at any point in the day – whatever works for you.

HOW DO I DO IT?

One session looks as follows:

HIIT round 1 / GVT round 1 / HIIT round 2 / GVT round 2

> *YOU NOT ONLY BURN CALORIES DURING THE WORKOUT BUT YOU ALSO BURN CALORIES FOR HOURS POST-WORKOUT*

1.   Pick any HIIT exercise and do 6 sets of 30 seconds with a 45-second rest between each set.
2.   Rest for 2 minutes.
3.   Begin GVT round 1. Do 10 sets of 10 reps, keeping the weight the same. Always keep a strict rest period of 60 seconds between each set.
4.   Perform another HIIT exercise for round 2: 6 sets of 30 seconds with a 45-second rest between each set.
5.   Rest for 2 minutes.
6.   Finally, on to GVT round 2. Do 10 sets of 10 reps, keeping the weight the same, with 60 seconds' rest between each set.
7.   Stretch and cool down.

HIIT EXERCISES

You can use any of these ideas for your HIIT rounds. You can repeat the same move for all sets or use a combination to form a circuit. Remember, the key here is to work your ass off for 30 seconds and then rest for 45 seconds and repeat that 6 times.

- Running on the spot
- Burpees
- Mountain climbers
- Running on the spot with punches
- Star jumps
- Tuck jumps

You can also perform your HIIT exercises on cardio equipment such as:

- Rowing machine
- Cross-trainer
- Exercise bike
- Treadmill
- Versa climber
- Boxing bag
- Battle ropes

WARM UP

Always carry out an exercise-specific warm up before starting your session. For example, if you are going to work your legs, I recommend doing some lunges and slow squats before picking up any weights. The aim is to warm up your muscles and joints so they're prepared for the exercise they're about to perform. This is really important to prevent injuries and ensure you get the most out of your workout, so please don't skip it!

> **Rest days are essential for muscle growth and recovery and will enhance your results**

PICK YOUR HIIT

**Choose from any of the following
6 exercises to build into your session**

/////////////////////////

HIIT option
1. Running on the spot

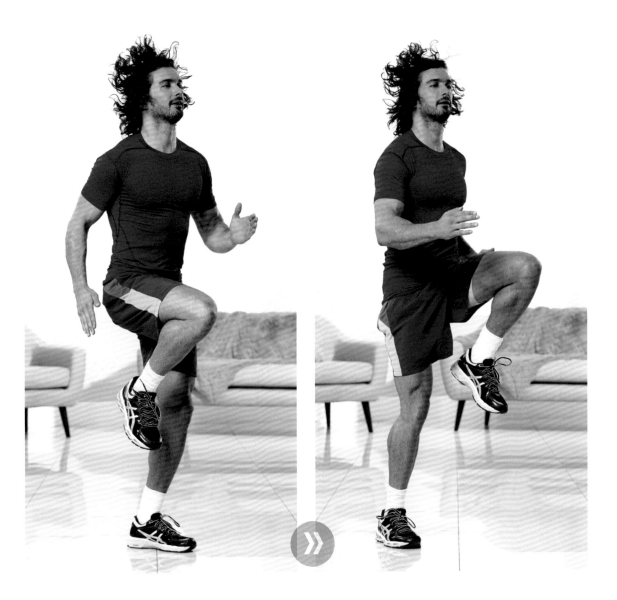

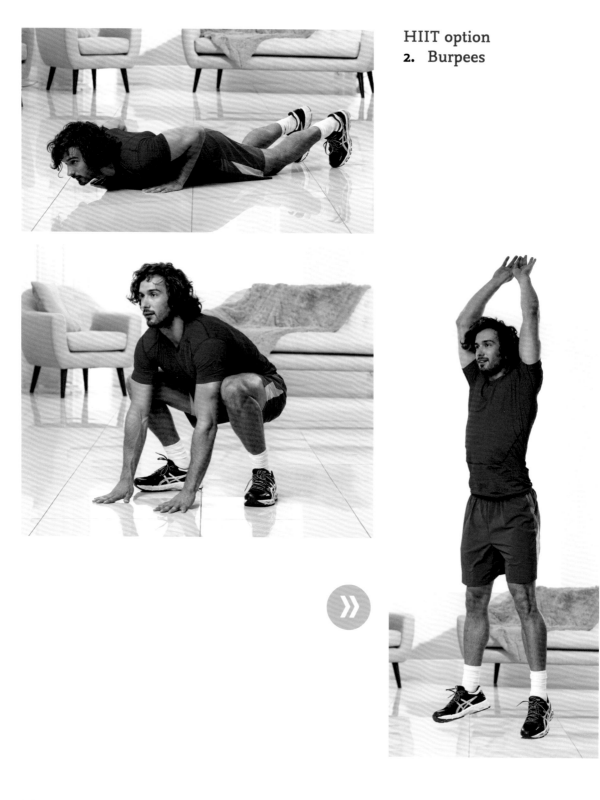

HIIT option
2. Burpees

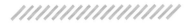

HIIT option
3. Mountain climbers

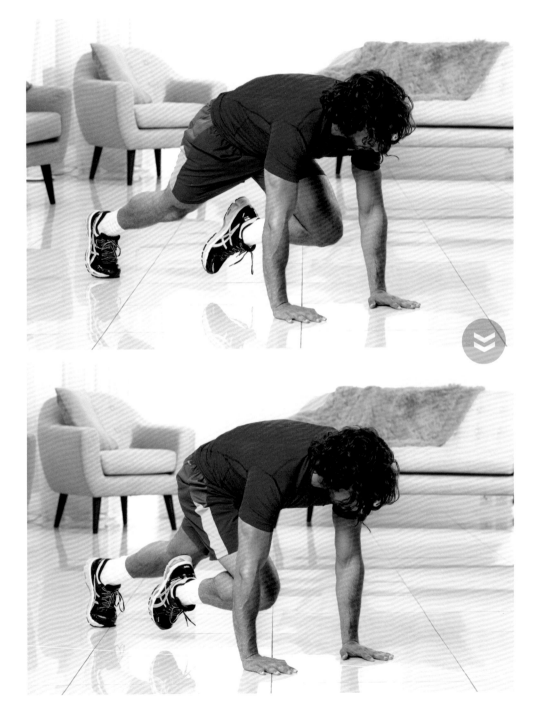

HIIT option
4. Running on the spot with punches

HIIT option
5. Star jumps

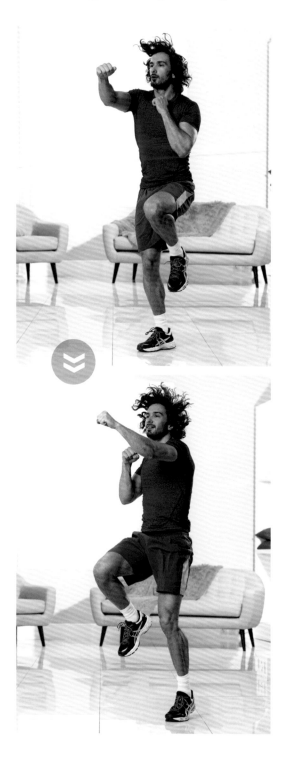

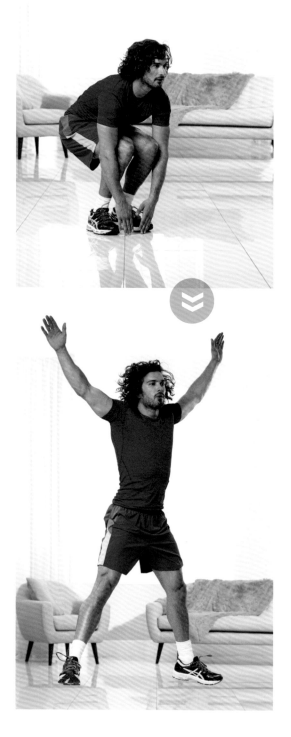

HIIT option
6. Tuck jumps

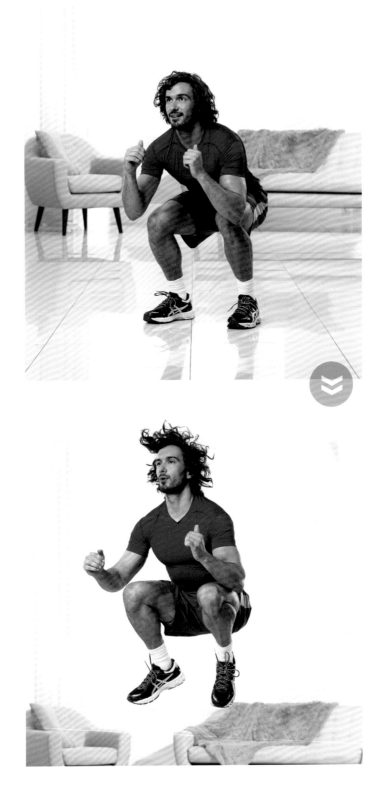

SESSION 1: ARMS (BICEPS AND TRICEPS)

Training description	Guidelines
HIIT round 1	6 sets of 30 seconds with a 45-second rest between sets (see HIIT exercises for ideas) Rest 2 minutes
GVT – biceps	Choose ONE of the following and perform 10 sets of 10 reps 1. Barbell curls 2. Hammer curls with dumbbells
HIIT round 2	6 sets of 30 seconds with a 45-second rest between sets (see HIIT exercises for ideas) Rest 2 minutes
GVT – triceps	Choose ONE of the following and perform 10 sets of 10 reps 1. Barbell skull crushers 2. Tricep kick-backs

1. Barbell curls

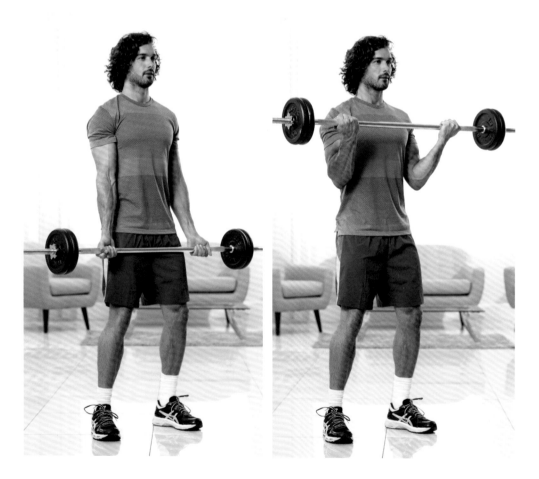

2. Hammer curls with dumbbells

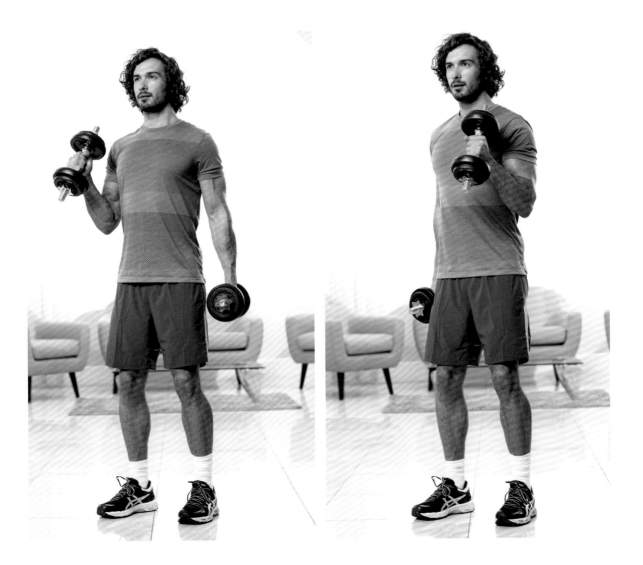

1. Barbell skull crushers

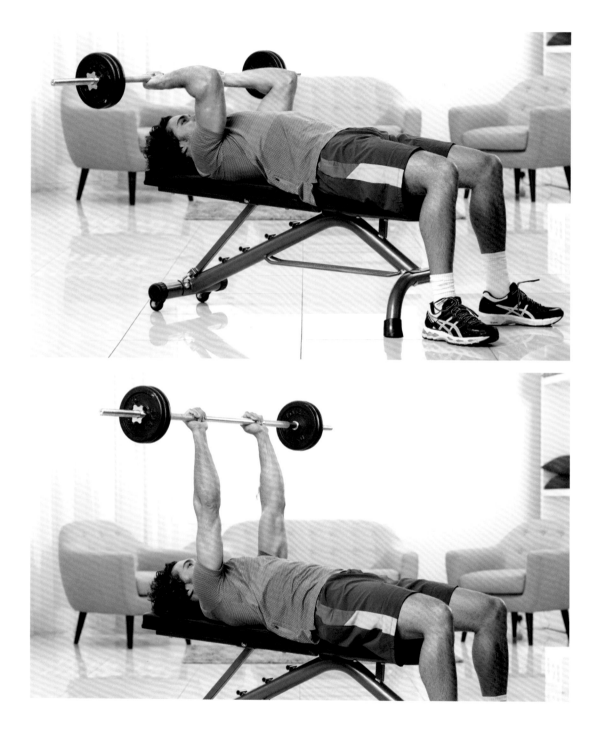

2. Tricep kick-backs

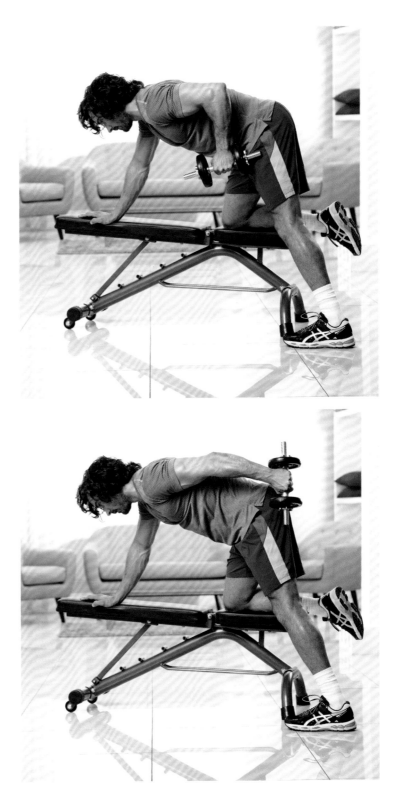

SESSION 2: CHEST AND BACK

Training description	Guidelines
HIIT round 1	6 sets of 30 seconds with a 45-second rest between sets (see HIIT exercises for ideas) Rest 2 minutes
GVT – chest	Choose ONE of the following and perform 10 sets of 10 reps 1. Barbell bench press 2. Dumbbell chest press
HIIT round 2	6 sets of 30 seconds with a 45-second rest between sets (see HIIT exercises for ideas) Rest 2 minutes
GVT – back	Choose ONE of the following and perform 10 sets of 10 reps 1. Single arm dumbbell rows 2. Bent-over barbell rows

1. Barbell bench press

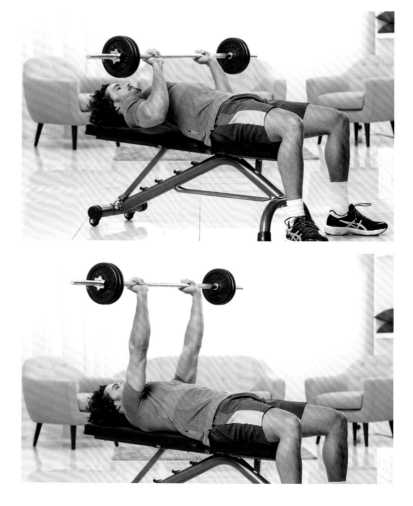

2. Dumbbell chest press

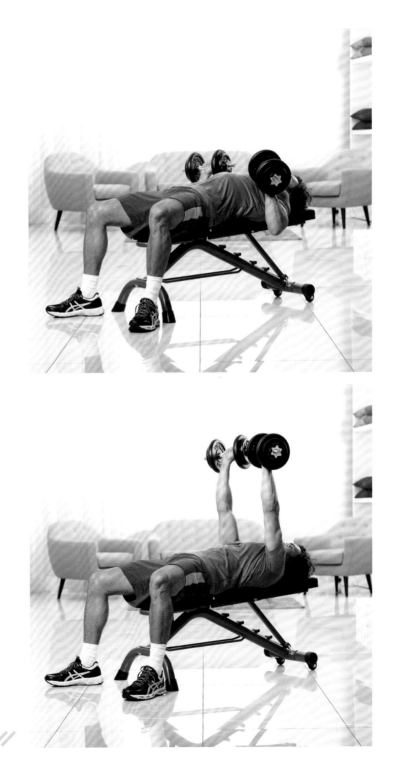

1. Single arm dumbbell rows

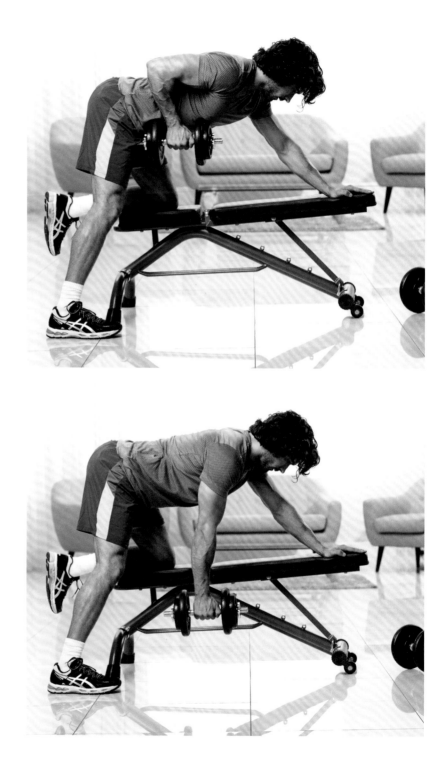

2. Bent-over
barbell rows

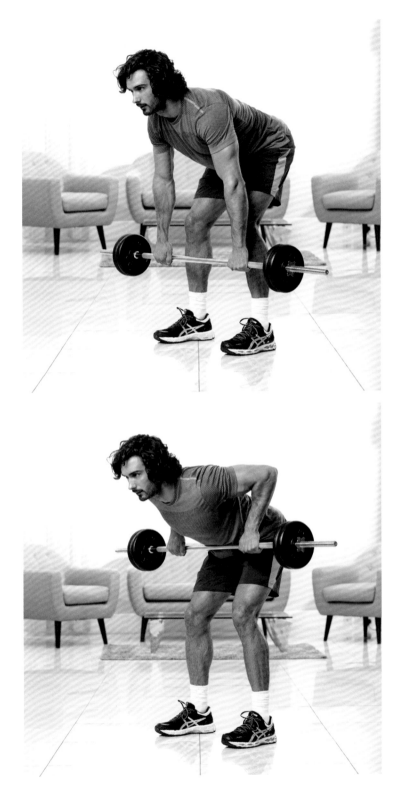

SESSION 3: LEGS (AND GLUTES)

Training description	Guidelines
HIIT round 1	6 sets of 30 seconds with a 45-second rest between sets (see HIIT exercises for ideas) │ Rest 2 minutes
GVT – legs	Choose ONE of the following and perform 10 sets of 10 reps 1. Barbell squats 2. Dumbbell squats
HIIT round 2	6 sets of 30 seconds with a 45-second rest between sets (see HIIT exercises for ideas) │ Rest 2 minutes
GVT – legs	Choose ONE of the following and perform 10 sets of 10 reps 1. Dumbbell lunges 2. Romanian deadlifts

1. Barbell squats

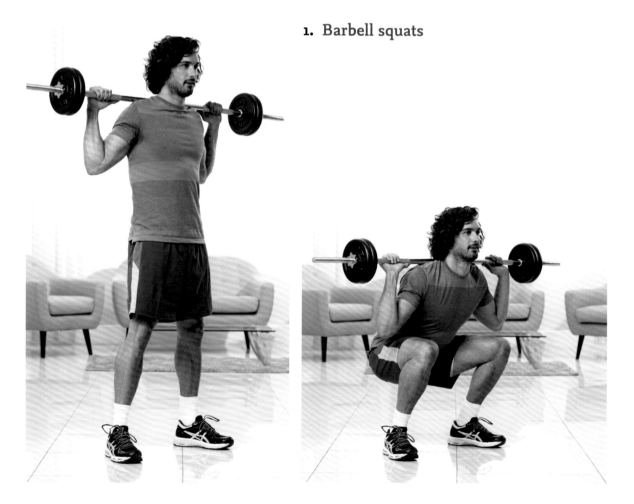

2. Dumbbell squats

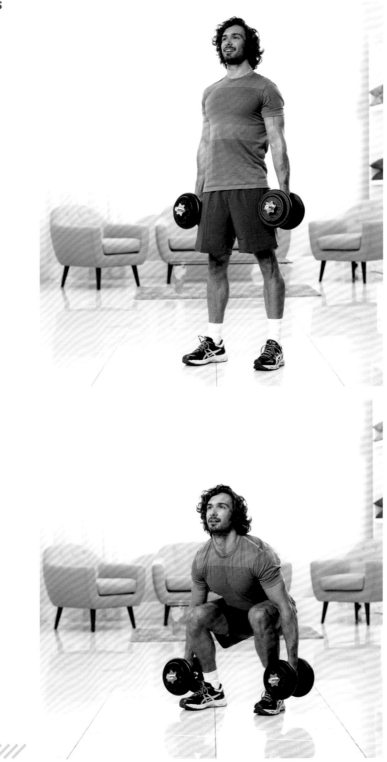

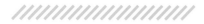

1. Dumbbell lunges

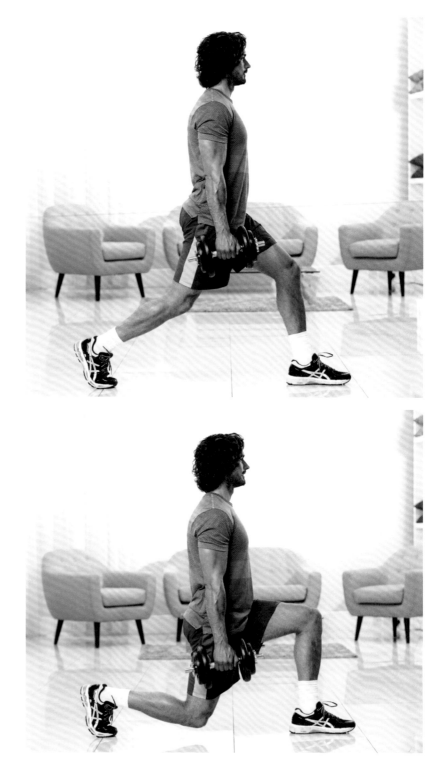

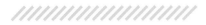

2. Romanian deadlifts

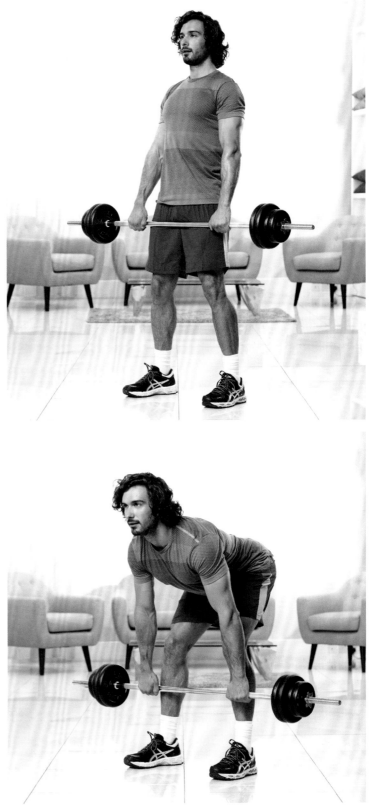

SESSION 4: SHOULDERS

Training description	Guidelines
HIIT round 1	6 sets of 30 seconds with a 45-second rest between sets (see HIIT exercises for ideas) | Rest 2 minutes
GVT – shoulders	Choose ONE of the following and perform 10 sets of 10 reps 1. Seated dumbbell shoulder press 2. Seated barbell shoulder press
HIIT round 2	6 sets of 30 seconds with a 45-second rest between sets (see HIIT exercises for ideas) | Rest 2 minutes
GVT – shoulders	Choose ONE of the following and perform 10 sets of 10 reps 1. Dumbbell lateral raises 2. Dumbbell frontal raises

1. Seated dumbbell shoulder press

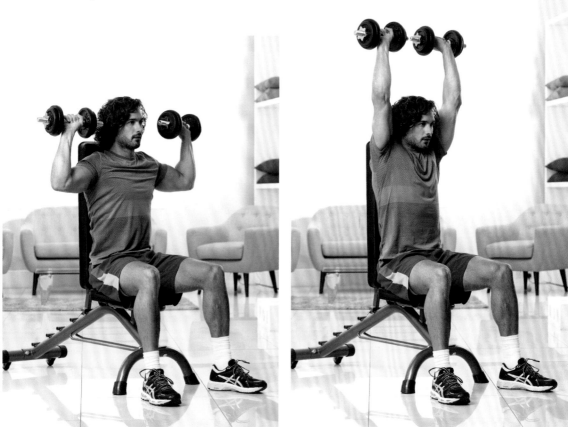

2. Seated barbell shoulder press

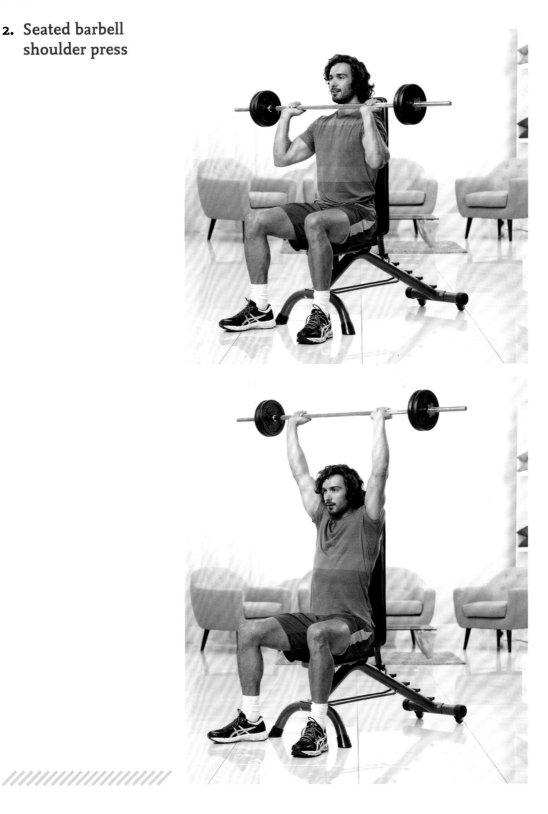

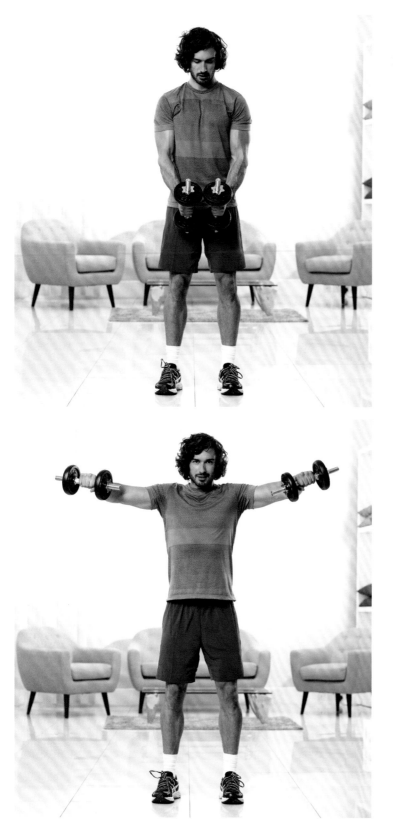

1. Dumbbell
lateral raises

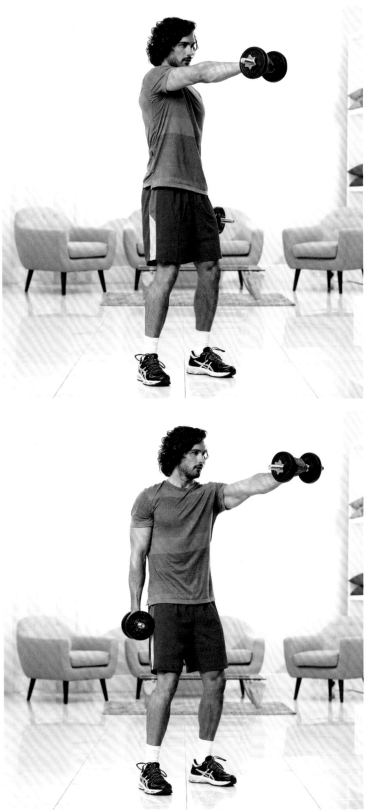

2. Dumbbell
frontal raises

COOL DOWN AND RECOVERY

//

After your workouts you may experience something called DOMS. This stands for delayed onset muscle soreness and can last between 24 and 72 hours. It can result in aching and stiffness due to muscle tissue damage. But don't worry, it's a sign you've worked hard and your muscles will quickly adapt by growing stronger, so it won't happen every time you train.

You can prevent the symptoms by gradually increasing the weights you use, rather than steaming in like Arnie and trying to lift the heaviest weights you can find. Start the programme with lighter weights to prime your body for the exercises, then each week you can slightly increase them.

After you finish a workout, be sure to do some stretching and mobility work. This could include yoga or Pilates exercises to ensure your joints stay mobile and your muscles remain flexible. This will keep your muscles nice and lean, improve your posture and reduce the risk of injury.

JOE'S POST-WORKOUT PROTEIN SHAKE

INGREDIENTS

1 scoop (30g) vanilla
  protein powder
15g honey
100g baby spinach leaves
handful of ice cubes

As you can see on page 26, I always have a protein shake with honey immediately after I train – it's great for muscle repair.

METHOD

Throw everything into a blender with a good splash of water and blitz until smooth.

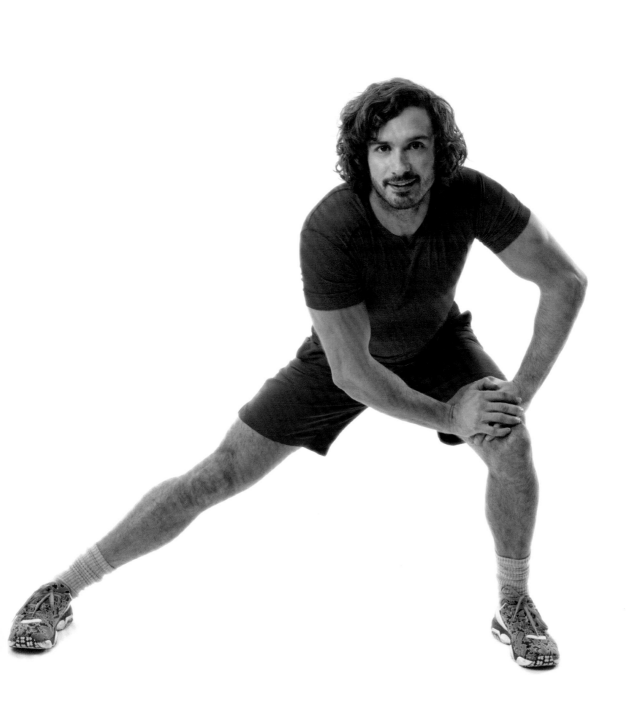

MY LEAN
WINNERS

7

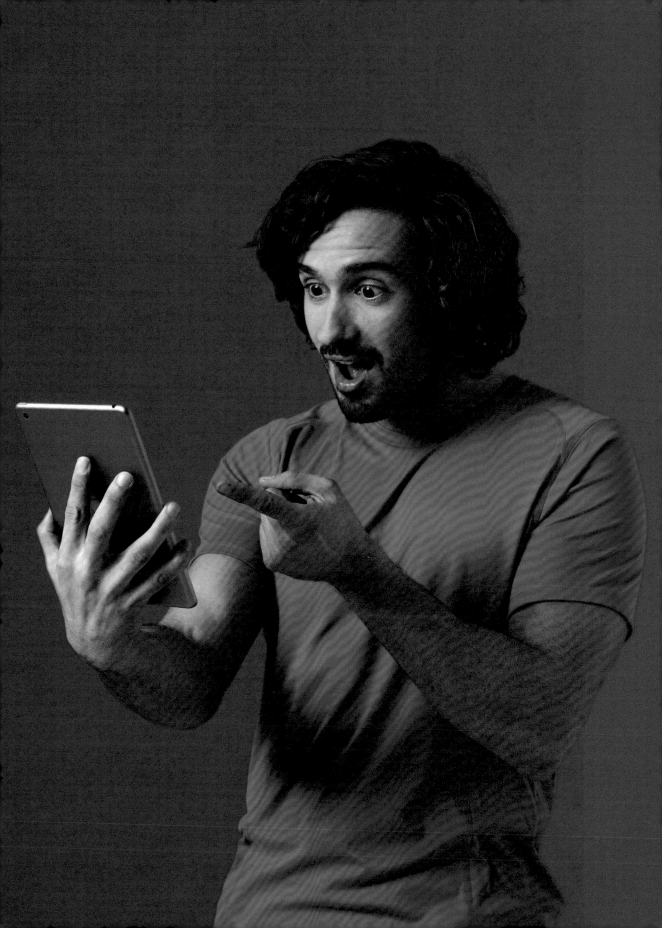

MY LEAN
WINNERS

///

This is one of my favourite sections of the book, where I can show you some of the most inspiring transformations from around the world. I don't get to meet my clients, as the plan and coaching are all delivered online, but each month they send in their progress pictures along with a written testimonial.

This is where I get to see the real impact my plan is having on people of all ages, shapes and sizes. Each client has a different story and works hard to overcome their own obstacles to get fitter, leaner and stronger.

I work with clients suffering from IBS, underactive thyroid glands, PCOS (polycystic ovary syndrome), diabetes, eating disorders and many other conditions, to improve their health. Some clients have been struggling on low-calorie diets for years and my plan rescues them from this because it teaches them how to fuel their bodies once and for all.

I've included a few transformations in this book (for privacy reasons I have omitted faces and @names) but if you want to see thousands more, check out the Transformations gallery at thebodycoach.co.uk.

❛ I have learned so much about nutrition and what my body needs ❜

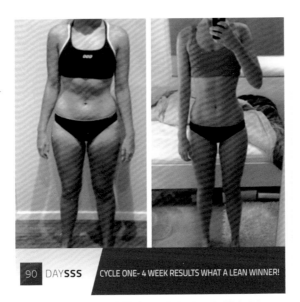

90 **DAYSSS** CYCLE ONE- 4 WEEK RESULTS WHAT A LEAN WINNER!

★ 'I have never been able to stick to anything like this: there were times when I would be at the gym twice a day, morning and night, with no idea how to fuel my body properly and definitely not seeing any results, then would go for weeks without doing anything at all because I'd lost motivation. I had no idea what nutrition my body needed and was almost punishing it with the amount of exercise and lack of food. Through the plan I have learned so much about nutrition and what my body needs. The HIIT is great – I now exercise for 25 minutes, it's literally a pre-shower routine, and I am eating more than I ever have in my life! The food is full of flavour and there's SO MUCH OF IT! The motivation comes from feeling the way you do on the plan. I still had dinners out and the odd naughty treat but was always ready to get back on it and smash out a HIIT session the next day, and was more informed in choosing healthier options eating out. This isn't a diet, it's a lifestyle change. You will 100 per cent not regret it. There are so many recipes to suit anyone's food preferences and the exercise fits into the day so easily. I can't wait for cycle two – seeing my pictures is so motivating and feeling this healthy for the first time in so long means I will never go back to the way I was before.'
Alexandra

‟ This has been a massive learning curve and one that I have really embraced and enjoyed „

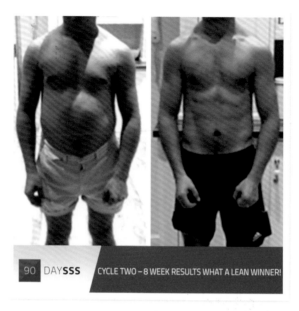

90 **DAYSSS** CYCLE TWO – 8 WEEK RESULTS WHAT A LEAN WINNER!

★ 'This has been a massive learning curve and one that I have really embraced and enjoyed. I have always been pretty sporty, from football and jiu jitsu to golf and running. However, I have never looked at my diet and what I'm eating (even though I knew it wasn't the best to say the least). This has given me the opportunity to experiment with home cooking, which again is not something I have done too much of in the past. I have also learned a lot more about the day-to-day intake of foods and drinks. As an example, when I was buying oats the other day I found myself looking at the sugar levels of different brands, which is definitely something I never thought I would say, let alone do. Everyone I know who has started or finished the Body Coach has become immersed within the programme, and like others I have found myself talking about it more often and not only to family and friends. This has truly been the start of a life-changing couple of months.' Stephan

❛I loved the weights, loved the food and loved how I felt ❜

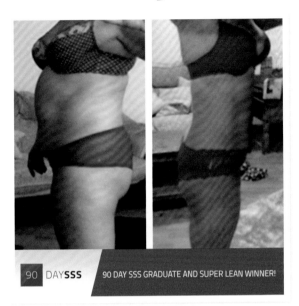

90 DAY**SSS** · 90 DAY SSS GRADUATE AND SUPER LEAN WINNER!

★ 'I can't quite believe how far I've come until I take my photos at the end of each cycle. I am a 50-year-old woman who has been on some kind of diet for 35 years! I absolutely loved cycle three. I started to see fat loss and muscle definition; I loved the weights, loved the food and loved how I felt. Fit, strong and in control. I will never ever go back to the way I was. I couldn't have done this without the forums on Facebook full of lovely leanies who give endless support and advice. And of course Joe, I am so utterly grateful for this plan, it really changed my life.' Kay

❝ I've learned so much about the way I should fuel my body ❞

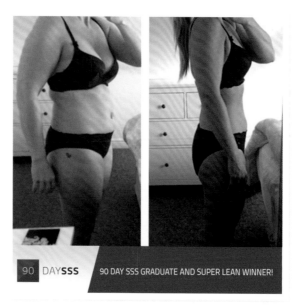

90 DAY**SSS**   90 DAY SSS GRADUATE AND SUPER LEAN WINNER!

★ 'I signed up for the plan after seeing the excellent results my friend got from it and from following people's progress on Facebook. I found the plan challenging but had faith in it and there was no way I was quitting after all the hard work and measuring of ingredients. I'd have kicked myself not to see it through to the end! I had my moments (a minor breakdown after trying to measure out curry portions went wrong!) but on the whole I stuck to it and persevered. The plan paid off, it does what it says on the tin. I've learned so much about the way I should fuel my body. Big thanks to Joe and his team of coaches.' Lynsey

This plan has really opened my eyes and is exactly what I needed to improve my relationship with food

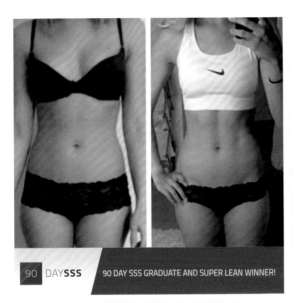

90 DAYSSS — 90 DAY SSS GRADUATE AND SUPER LEAN WINNER!

★ 'I always thought I maintained a healthy and balanced lifestyle, but this plan has really opened my eyes and is exactly what I needed to improve my relationship with food. Three months ago I was counting almost every calorie I ate and skipping meals or undereating if I felt I'd "over-indulged". I'd then partner this with a 4-mile run 3–4 times a week and was consistently disappointed when I never noticed any change in my body shape. Joe's plan has taught me the fundamental importance of food and how it fuels your body for exercise. Although initially it was a little tough, since starting the plan I haven't once thought about the number of calories I'm eating because, to put it simply, my body needed them!' Alix

' Every day, I see changes – more importantly, I feel those changes '

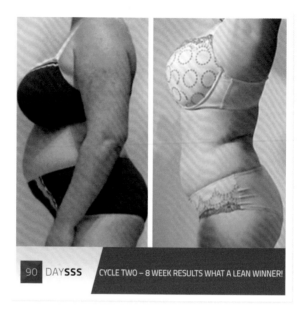

90 **DAY**SSS CYCLE TWO – 8 WEEK RESULTS WHAT A LEAN WINNER!

★ 'I'm fascinated by how the process works, and cannot get my head around it. When you say the fat melts, you're not kidding are you?! Every day, I see changes – more importantly, I feel those changes. I was hardly a vociferous weigh-inner before, but ignoring the scales (and indeed the tape measure, or camera) for a month at a time means that you have a day when you feel proud, and strong, and like you've really achieved and there's nothing to take it away from you. It all belongs to you. Looking back at me is a map of my journey, the determination and possibility in the changing landscape of my body.' Ruth

> **I'm sleeping so much better now ... I feel so much happier in myself as well as healthy**

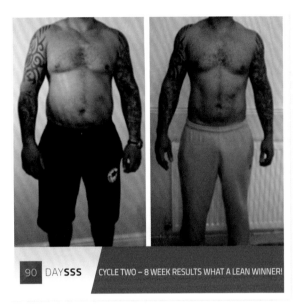

90 DAY**SSS**   CYCLE TWO – 8 WEEK RESULTS WHAT A LEAN WINNER!

★ 'I watched other people making great progress, so I knew I could do it – anyone can! I really enjoyed the introduction of weight training. I've always used the gym for weights but never cardio, so both together is fantastic, even more so when you know eating the right foods afterwards will help you get the most from doing it, making it all the more worthwhile. And finally, I'm sleeping so much better now. I work permanent nights so sleep is very important to me. I feel so much happier in myself as well as healthy. I feel solid and not flabby and I'm seeing so much more definition, #LEAN!!!!!! And my hips are the same size as my waist! Fantastic.' Ross

LEAN IN 15
HEROES

//

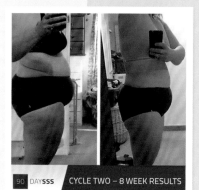

90 DAYSSS CYCLE TWO – 8 WEEK RESULTS

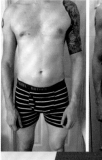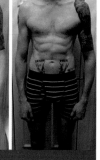

90 DAYSSS 90 DAY SSS GRADUATE

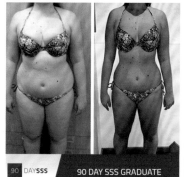

90 DAYSSS 90 DAY SSS GRADUATE

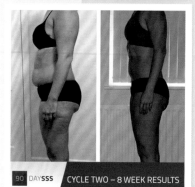

90 DAYSSS CYCLE TWO – 8 WEEK RESULTS

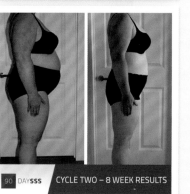

90 DAYSSS CYCLE TWO – 8 WEEK RESULTS

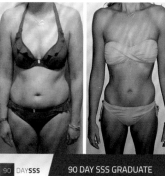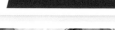

90 DAYSSS 90 DAY SSS GRADUATE

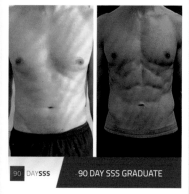

90 DAYSSS 90 DAY SSS GRADUATE

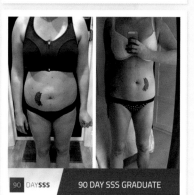

90 DAYSSS 90 DAY SSS GRADUATE

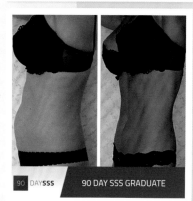

90 DAYSSS 90 DAY SSS GRADUATE

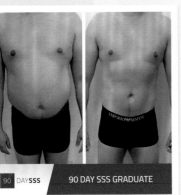

90 DAY SSS GRADUATE

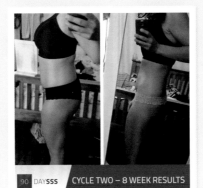

CYCLE TWO – 8 WEEK RESULTS

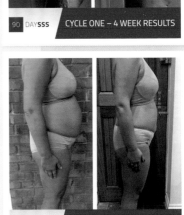

CYCLE ONE – 4 WEEK RESULTS

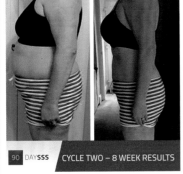

CYCLE TWO – 8 WEEK RESULTS

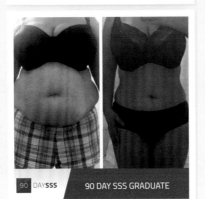

90 DAY SSS GRADUATE

CYCLE TWO – 8 WEEK RESULTS

CYCLE TWO – 8 WEEK RESULTS

CYCLE TWO – 8 WEEK RESULTS

CYCLE ONE – 4 WEEK RESULTS

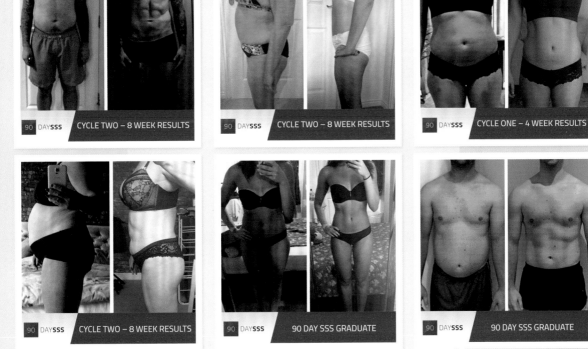

CYCLE TWO – 8 WEEK RESULTS

90 DAY SSS GRADUATE

90 DAY SSS GRADUATE

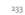

INDEX

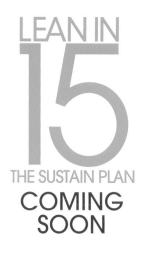

LEAN IN
15
THE SUSTAIN PLAN
COMING SOON

ACKNOWLEDGEMENTS

I would like to start by thanking all the lean winners who have ever signed up to my 90 Day Shift, Shape and Sustain Plan. I would also like to thank all my support coach heroes who have helped me help so many people get fitter and healthier. With your help I truly believe we will change the fat-loss and diet industry forever.

I also want to thank my two amazing editors Carole and Olivia for helping me create this book and for being so patient when I kept missing my deadlines. Guilty, your honour.

Thank you to my manager Bev, who from the start believed in me and made me set bigger goals and take bigger action.

And finally, a big shout-out to all my friends and family who love and encourage me in my mission to get the world lean.

See you in December for *Lean in 15*, volume 3 – *The Sustain Plan*.

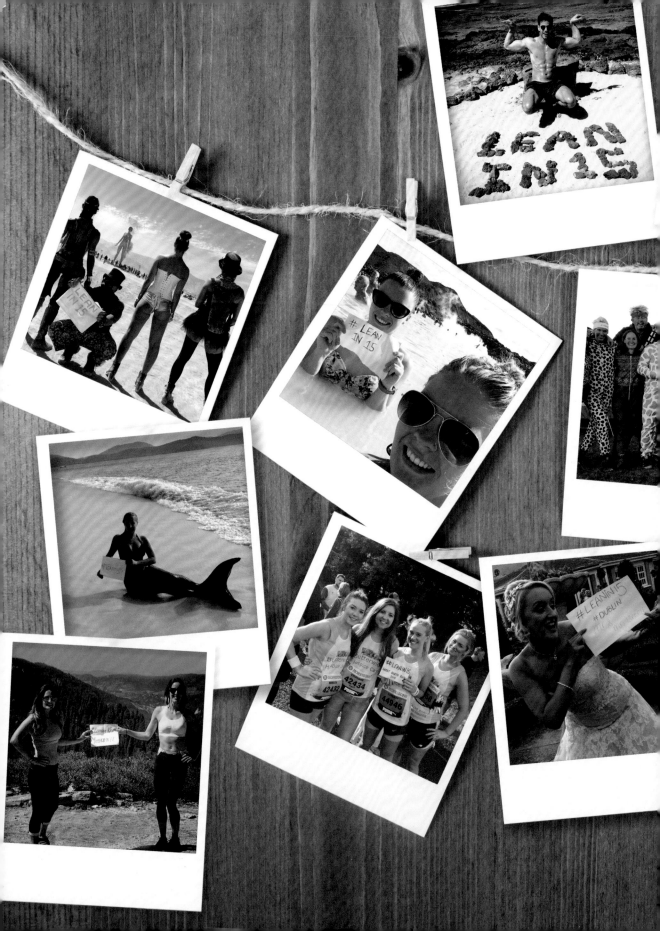

LEAN IN 15 AROUND THE WORLD

Tag your own pictures from around the world with the hashtag #Leanin15

KEEP IN TOUCH:

- For more recipes follow me on Facebook, Instagram and Twitter (@thebodycoach)
- Tag your meals and progress pictures with the hashtag #Leanin15
- For more workout videos check out my YouTube channel – The Body Coach TV

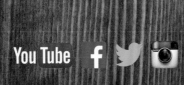

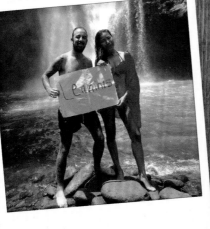

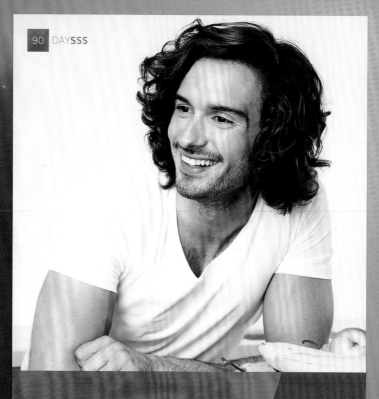

90 DAY**SSS**

To get your tailored plan and
start your transformation visit
www.thebodycoach.co.uk